TIM NOAKES
THE QUIET
MAVERICK

TIM NOAKES
THE QUIET
MAVERICK

DARYL ILBURY

PENGUIN BOOKS

Published by Penguin Books
an imprint of Penguin Random House South Africa (Pty) Ltd
Reg. No. 1953/000441/07
The Estuaries No. 4, Oxbow Crescent, Century Avenue, Century City, 7441
PO Box 1144, Cape Town, 8000, South Africa
www.penguinrandomhouse.co.za

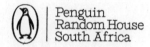

Penguin
Random House
South Africa

First published 2017

1 3 5 7 9 10 8 6 4 2

Publication © Penguin Random House 2017
Text © Daryl Ilbury 2017

Cover photograph © Sofia Dadourian

PUBLISHER: Marlene Fryer
MANAGING EDITOR: Ronel Richter-Herbert
EDITOR: Bronwen Maynier
PROOFREADER: Ronel Richter-Herbert
COVER DESIGN: Sean Robertson
TEXT DESIGN: Ryan Africa
TYPESETTING: Monique van den Berg

Set in 11.5 pt on 16 pt Minion

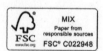

Printed by **novus print**, a Novus Holdings company

MIX
Paper from
responsible sources
FSC
www.fsc.org FSC® C022948

This book is printed on FSC® certified and controlled sources.
FSC (Forest Stewardship Council®) is an independent, international,
non-governmental organization. Its aim is to support environmentally sustainable,
socially and economically responsible global forest management.

ISBN 978 1 7760 9137 9 (print)
ISBN 978 1 7760 9138 6 (ePub)

For Chants, Rox and Mitch — my emotional macronutrients 2019-04-09

Contents

Author's note ix

1. Introduction: The Great Centenary Debate 1
2. 'Newton, we have a problem': The uncomfortable
   truth about science and human nature 14
3. When science drops the ball: The uncomfortable
   truth about the nature of science 32
4. A maverick in the ear: Noakes on the sidelines 54
5. Noakes on Noakes 73
6. Prometheus rejected: Science in the media 85
7. Human nutrition: It's not a soundbite, people! 110
8. The trial 136
9. Disruption and reflection 173

Bibliography 199

Author's note

My hope is that this book is not what you expect it to be; it must be more than that. It is inspired by a maxim in science journalism: content is king, context is King Kong. Briefly, this means that while examining the facts may provide valuable information, standing back to see the big picture encourages a far more compelling beast to emerge.

This book is not just about Tim Noakes. It's also about you, and your relationship with science, the media and with what you eat. More importantly, it's about the media's relationship with science, and how you fit into it. This is important because it determines how you interpret what is playing out in science and the impact you can have.

It's also not an homage to Tim Noakes. This book asks some very tough questions. It explores some of the criticisms levelled against him and listens to some of those quite vocal in challenging him. But it also gives a voice to those who have worked intimately with him to help explain why he does what he does and what drives him. I leave it up to you to make up your own mind about him.

This book is also not all about the Health Professions Council of South Africa (HPCSA) hearing against Noakes, for two reasons: firstly, at the time of its writing, the hearing was still in progress, and, secondly, the hearing deserves its own book – it had so many plots, subplots, and twists and turns. No, the focus of this book is the backstory – the events and conditions that laid the foundation for the hearing. Having said that, I have covered what I think are key components to the hearing, and these make up the largest chapter.

I could have provided you with a simple outcome or answer as to whether what Noakes says about nutrition is right or wrong, but that would have insulted your intelligence. It also would not have been much fun. Instead, I have sewn threads throughout the book, within the different layers of what is a very complex issue, leaving you to tie them together to see that big picture. I have reserved judgement, but I admit to including subtle clues as to how I feel about certain elements of the topic under discussion. Those who know me from my days on radio will no doubt find that familiar.

This is also not a straightforward book about science. It is partly a personal journey to understand what makes Tim Noakes tick. I have therefore had to balance the discipline demanded of science journalism with the creative licence of science writing. The result, I hope, is a story that is both rigorous and enjoyable, but with a more conversational narrative. For that you can blame over 25 years in radio and the instinct to write for the ear. Hopefully this has created the impression that you are, at times, sitting in the room with Tim Noakes.

I have assumed that the average reader is not a specialist in human nutrition, and therefore have attempted to explain some of the technicalities about the science of the topic. This has demanded a degree of simplification. This always risks irking specialists, especially those with a more pedant temperament. If you are a specialist in the respective sections I cover, feel free to skip over them. I won't take it personally.

If parts of the story seem familiar, there's a reason for that. In October 2012 I was asked by Anton Harber to write a 10 000-word book about Tim Noakes for his fledgling publishing company Mampoer Shorts (the details are in Chapter 1). I titled it *The Quiet Maverick*, but the editors decided on another title: *Tim Noakes Chews the Fat*. It sold well for Mampoer; very well, in fact, but it was not sufficient to save the company, which closed in August 2014. They returned the publishing rights to me, and it seemed the story would remain largely unknown to all but the handful that had read it.

Luckily, one of those was Marlene Fryer of Penguin Random House. When I contacted her in March 2015 with the idea of publishing a selection from my varied newspaper and magazine columns, Marlene immediately arranged a meeting, and asked me to write for her. The ink wasn't even dry on my first book for her, *A Fox's Tale*, when Marlene asked, 'So what's next?' By them the HPCSA hearing against Tim Noakes was in full swing and I was sitting with the rights to the ebook and a trove of information about him had not been able to use. 'How about a book on Tim Noakes?' Marlene agreed without hesitation; the result is now in your hands.

It would not have been possible without the input, patience and support of a number of people. Firstly, all the contributors and those I interviewed, primarily Tim Noakes, who made himself available for interviews, answered all my questions, provided access to his archives and not once asked to check what I was writing – that's rare for a scientist. Secondly, all my family, and especially my wife Chantell, who is my fiercest critic and primary grounding force. She allowed me the space and time to write, and forgave me for nodding and shaking my head at the seemingly correct times when she was talking to me, knowing all along my mind was 'in writing mode' and not listening to a word she was

2019-04-09
20190409

saying. To the team at Penguin Random House, especially my publisher Marlene Fryer, for believing in me, my managing editor Ronel Richter-Herbert for keeping me in focus and cracking the whip, and my publicist Surita Joubert for somehow bending space and time.

2019-04-09

And finally, a special thank you to Mrs Roberts, my Grade 11 English teacher who, calling me to her desk one day to critique an essay I had written, titled 'No More Hiroshimas', tapped my book with her finger, looked up at me, smiled and said, 'You know, you could be a writer one day.'

DARYL ILBURY
CAPE TOWN
MARCH 2017

Chapter 1

Introduction:
The Great Centenary Debate

It is almost impossible to hate Tim Noakes. A boyish, almost 2019-04-09
goofy smile is never far from his face; he is generally mild man-
nered to the point of reticence in social situations; and to the best
of my knowledge, he has never so much as wished anyone any
harm. In fact, stories abound of his going out of his way to help
those who have turned to him for guidance. Still, there was no
mistaking the venom in the air when he stepped up to address
colleagues, friends and fellow academics at the University of Cape
Town (UCT) on the evening of 6 December 2012.

Under the interrogative glare of the TV lights, Noakes turned
to face a packed lecture theatre heaving with people wearing
condemnatory frowns (the academic equivalent of bared teeth),
hunched forward, ready to scrutinise his every word. He may as
well have been blindfolded with a target pinned to his chest.

The occasion was a debate. But this was no typical intellectual parley over academic minutiae. This was going to get nasty,
because the honour of an entire discipline within the health
sciences had been challenged.

At the time, all this was lost on me. I was there, to a degree, in desperation. A few months earlier I had graduated from City, University of London with a master's degree in science journalism attenuated by the sobering realisation that science journalists around the world were among the first line of specialists being culled by media organisations facing crippling budget constraints. I had returned to Cape Town to find that there were three areas where science was still in the papers: technology, the environment and health (soon to be lumped together with fashion and make-up tips under the more attractive heading 'lifestyle').

I decided to focus on health because it seemed the best avenue for work. It certainly was not the easiest option – it wasn't my area of interest – but I figured I would learn along the way. I became a regular writer for the *Business Day* weekly *Health News* supplement, as well as other titles, and felt secure that perhaps, just perhaps, the storm clouds over science journalism in South Africa would dissipate.

I was wrong. By the time Tim Noakes stood up to address that crowd, my job as a science journalist was disappearing. The previous week I had been told that *Business Day* was closing the *Health News* supplement. The decision was blamed on budget constraints that didn't seem to bother the motoring supplement – a case of torque being more important than testicular cancer, I mused. I had just completed a piece about South African rugby hero Tendai 'Beast' Mtawarira's battle with atrial fibrillation and it looked like it wasn't going to go anywhere. And things were to get worse. Little did I know, sitting there at UCT, that the very next day Colin Roopnarain of the *Sunday Tribune* magazine supplement would send me a mail telling me that due to 'major budget cuts' the magazine was culling all external contributors.

I had been a regular columnist for the *Sunday Tribune* for two and a half years, writing about the rather uncomfortable relationship South Africans had with science. Ironically, the news came in the same week that basic education minister Angie Motshekga announced, at the release of the annual national assessment results, that the average score in maths for Grade 9 learners (approximately 14 years of age) was 13 per cent. No, that is not a typo; that really is 13 per cent. It was also the same week that Times Media public editor Joe Latakgomo published an opinion piece saying it should be the press's responsibility to remove from their pages personal ads from people masquerading as doctors who offer (to a very willing and receptive consumer) a combined portfolio of services normally including penis enlargement, cleaning dirty money, fixing broken marriages and winning the lottery.

There was a ray of hope, though. I had just signed a contract with Mampoer Shorts, the e-publishing venture of Anton Harber, Professor of Journalism at the University of the Witwatersrand. His idea was for short, punchy books penned by experienced writers. I had contacted him months earlier with my idea for an independent science desk that would collate and provide stories to various news titles. It was an unconventional, if somewhat naive, idea that was doomed from the start, but it did earn me an email from Anton with the invitation to write something about Professor Tim Noakes and his controversial reversal of opinion on carbohydrates. The brief from Anton was the following: find out if he's a flip-flopper, or an evidence-based scientist.

That's why I was waiting for Noakes to speak, notepad and pen ready, voice recorder charged. But don't think for a minute I was excited to be there. Truth be told, I had signed the contract with Mampoer Shorts with mixed feelings. I had little interest in sports science, Noakes's field of expertise, and the broader debate – nutrition – required a background in biology, something I had last studied at the age of 14. I had interviewed Noakes before for a *Business Day* piece in defence of the humble potato, which had become the bad boy on the veggie block. At that stage, it was going through what sugar is going through now – a sustained attack by self-styled health gurus who saw an opportunity in burgeoning waistlines and hysterical headlines to take potshots at their least favourite food. What really impressed my editor was that I had managed to get comment from a very busy Noakes, who proved to be pleasant, engaging and particularly interested in the angle of my story.

There was something else: in his response to my questions, Noakes had displayed an understanding of what a journalist looks for in an interview – clear, concise answers in easy-to-understand language. I thought if any scientist could provide an uncomplicated avenue into a highly complicated issue, it would be Noakes. I would be wrong.

As I sat, waiting for the protagonist of my project to start proceedings, I scanned through the notes I had scribbled beforehand. Those coming out fighting were two major heavyweights: in the one corner was Professor Tim Noakes, the Discovery Health Chair of Exercise and Sports Science and director of the MRC/UCT Research Unit for Exercise Science and Sports Medicine in the Department of Human Biology at UCT, and co-founder, with Springbok rugby legend Morné du Plessis, of the Sports Science Institute of South Africa.

In the other corner was Dr Jacques Rossouw, the former Professor of Medicine at Stellenbosch University and director of the Medical Research Council National Research Institute for Nutritional Diseases; past president of the South African Nutrition Society and Chair of the Scientific Advisory Committee to the Heart Foundation of Southern Africa; and now chief of the Women's Health Initiative Branch in the Division of Cardiovascular Sciences at the US National Heart, Lung, and Blood Institute, which is part of the National Institutes of Health (NIH).

Everyone knew Noakes; he was a darling of the media. However, for that he had earned the annoyance of many fellow scientists, who believed 'popularising' science risked stripping it of its accuracy, and that speaking to a media that flirted with tabloid sentiment meant that science was reduced to snippets of sensationalism. He also seemed to enjoy the media spotlight, a crime that was to later earn him the inglorious titles 'celebrity scientist' and 'rock star scientist'. He was also a specialist in sports science, which may have been closer to the heart of many South Africans, but only recently allowed into the hallowed halls of academia, and kept somewhat at arm's length until it was decided it had earned its place as a 'serious' science.

Despite that, Noakes had risen through the ranks of a highly competitive and uncompromising academia. He had done so through dogged hard work, with little pause for the unwritten protocols of conformity. It was fair to say that he had earned a mix of respect and rebuke.

Rossouw was unknown to me, and I think it would be fair to say unknown to most people outside of those in the room or who had studied medicine under his watch. But I gathered he was an academic's academic – restrained, somewhat stoical, but unreserved in his distrust of the media. He believed science was best kept to scientists, and he lived for the regulations that kept the centuries-old discipline of medical research on track. He was the exact opposite of Noakes, so there was an element of tension in the room.

There was something else stoking the levels of anticipation: the event, which was part of the celebrations attendant on the 100th anniversary of the health sciences faculty of the University of Cape Town, had been titled 'The Great Centenary Debate'. A little theatrical, I thought, but Noakes was there to present an argument that even with my patchy knowledge of matters of

5

2019-04-09

health was a clear challenge to medical convention. It was titled: 'Cholesterol is not an important factor for heart disease and current dietary recommendations do even more harm than good'. Not very 'sporty', I remember thinking. Granted, he had been making a name for himself as a popular advocate for eschewing all things carbohydrate, a complete flip on the policy of 'carbo-loading' he had championed in *Lore of Running*, the so-called runner's bible he had authored in 1985 – but 'cholesterol'? Why was he now talking about cholesterol? I thought it a little off-point for a sports scientist, but I had no idea of the drama that he was about to unfold. This was not Noakes typically 'meddling', as was often the accusation by those whose thinking he challenged; he was doing nothing less than throwing down a gauntlet at the feet of what he would refer to as nutritional 'dogma'.

Rossouw was there to provide evidence to underscore conventional wisdom, thereby supposedly correcting Noakes's research. But most attendees were hoping for more – that he would put Noakes back in his place, send him with tail between legs back to the sports field and away from the more serious field of human nutrition. They may have had a respect for Noakes the sports scientist, and were prepared to tip their hats to his international standing in this regard, but they believed he had now crossed the line and was out of play. They wanted him to pay the penalty for challenging everything they believed to be true and a central tenet to their entire discipline. Rossouw was going to give him a bloody nose; Noakes was going down. I didn't realise it at the time, but I had a ringside seat to what was expected to be Noakes's unequivocal comeuppance. Noakes suspected this going into the debate. He was to tell me later, 'It was a set-up.'

Noakes spoke first, and, in a style that has made him popular with the media, kept his argument as accessible as possible. He made no bones about his claim: 'I have to convince you that what you've been taught for the past 60 years is rubbish.'

Vintage Noakes, albeit a little alarming. I sensed those around me bristle. He used simple graphs and images, and peppered his argument with entertaining anecdotes and references to socio-political policies and associated sciences that have impacted on human nutrition. However, his message was clear and harsh: the commonly held belief that coronary heart disease (CHD) was caused by a high-fat diet was based on incomplete, and sometimes flimsy, research; and that despite the flimsiness of the evidence, the claim had penetrated the thinking of the medical profession so deeply as to be akin to blind faith. Even I felt a little disturbed; this was hard-hitting stuff. His secondary message was, if anything, even more provocative: that the dietary advice premised on this claim was doing more harm than good, because it was contribut-ing to the increase in levels of obesity and its associated illnesses.

He went on to say that whereas high levels of cholesterol were not an insignificant factor, one of the main culprits behind CHD, and hitherto seemingly ignored, was the insulin spikes that the body sometimes endures when it processes carbohydrates – chemical compounds, including sugars and starch found in cereals, breads, flour and sweets, which the body breaks down to produce glucose in order to fuel its cells. The hormone insulin is a critical component in the processing of carbohydrates; it helps 'open up' cells to accept the resultant glucose. By overloading on carbohydrates, the body could easily generate too much insulin, with health-threatening consequences. This, according to Noakes, is especially dangerous for people such as himself, who are 'insu-lin resistant' – a condition where muscle, fat and liver cells are unable to respond properly to insulin and thus cannot easily absorb glucose from the bloodstream. As a result, the body needs higher levels of insulin to help glucose enter cells. The overall metabolic effect of being insulin resistant is similar to when the body is unable to produce enough insulin: the result is a build-up of fat and the susceptibility to a portfolio of other complications, such as kidney failure, high blood pressure and CHD. It also dramatically opens up the path to a condition called 'pre-diabetic', in which blood sugar levels are higher than normal but not high enough for a diagnosis of diabetes. This can develop into type 2 diabetes.

His focus on this was very clear, and I distinctly remember writing down the term 'insulin resistance'. I had never heard of it before, despite a history of diabetes in my family that I was encouraged by my doctor to keep on my radar. My maternal grandfather had suffered from diabetes, and its impact on his life had been profound. He had both his legs amputated as a result of one of the many complications of this crippling disease: nerve damage and poor circulation in the feet and legs that encourage the growth of ulcers, resulting in untreatable tissue damage. His body never recovered, and he died shortly after the amputation. Noakes now had my attention.

Research, he went on to argue, has shown that diabetes is a disease growing in prevalence in South Africa, due to a significant degree to rising levels of obesity. This was something that few specialists could deny. It was also something that had been gaining traction in the media. It also wasn't just a South African problem. Stories were emerging from other Western media outlets that pointed towards a worrying upward trend in levels of obesity, and it wasn't just affecting adults – childhood obesity was on the rise, too.

There was something else that Noakes presented as a point of consent: most experts agree that obesity and a lack of physical activity can lead to insulin resistance; however, Noakes added that because insulin resistance can contribute to weight gain, the result can be a spiralling cycle of degenerating health. Furthermore, Noakes believed, insulin resistance is more prevalent than is commonly acknowledged. Making matters even worse, unlike fat in food, which is satiating and discourages binges or addictive eating, the insulin spikes resulting from carbohydrates can be addictive and encourage overeating. Fat was good, he said, and his solution for those who are sufferers of this condition was clear: a low-carbohydrate, high-protein and high-fat diet.

There was a problem: this is the exact opposite of traditional 'Western' nutritional guidelines that advocate a low-fat, high-carbohydrate diet. I knew others had tried to sound a warning cry against these guidelines, and the reaction by so-called established science had been swift and ruthless. Remember the fallout around the Atkins Diet?

That intrigued me. Disputes within science are a cornerstone of its strength. This may seem counter-intuitive, but science requires that what it believes to be evident should be robustly and continually challenged. There's a firm caveat: this should be done within the disciplined realms of academic research, preferably away from a reactive, largely scientifically illiterate, unquestioning populace under the sway of social media. This was one of the reasons for the fractious mood in the lecture room; there was a growing awareness of the potential impact – some may say 'damage' – of a man with Tim Noakes's experience and popular appeal in calling for the upending of established medical opinion. As he progressed through his presentation, heads shook slowly and a rising unease took hold.

Under pressure from the mediator watching the clock to wrap up his argument, Noakes delivered what he hoped was his *coup de grâce*: evidence buried within the data of a landmark and oft-quoted study as part of the Women's Health Initiative – a major 15-year research programme in the US designed to address the most common causes of death, disability and poor quality of life in postmenopausal women, namely cardiovascular disease, cancer and osteoporosis. More importantly for Noakes's argument, it was a study overseen by his challenger, Dr Rossouw. It supported Noakes's argument that a high-carbohydrate diet produced dangerous high-level spikes of insulin in those people with a predisposition towards diabetes. He then quoted Rossouw directly from his own summary of the study: '[This] shows that just reducing total fat intake does not go far enough to have an impact on heart disease.'

It was as if he had reached across and punched Rossouw in the chest. The audience recoiled. It was the closest Noakes had stepped towards personally confronting his challenger and labelling him an active agent in what Noakes saw as a conspiracy. It was perceived not so much as a shot across the bow as a direct hit. Being accused of inertia in the face of changing developments in science is not very nice. It happens – in a discipline where people spend decades pouring all their time and resources into understanding something, to have that overturned doesn't come without fight-back, and the inevitable damage to professional pride – but suggesting complicity in the cover-up of dodgy science is another thing altogether. Noakes seemed unapologetic.

Attention then turned to Rossouw and how he would address this apparently damning revelation. His opening remarks were an open admission that his presentation might seem a little dry: 'I'm not going to be half as entertaining as Tim.' Everyone laughed. At first it seemed a professional nod to Noakes's popular communicative style, but Rossouw made it clear what he really meant when he added, 'I'm also not going to touch on anecdotes, anthropology or agricultural policy. I will touch on associations, but I will only do so in general when you have meta-analyses with robust data.' It was a subtle but clear suggestion that Noakes's proposal lacked any scientific integrity, and an attempt to turn the quality of Noakes's presentation skills into an implicit weakness; to make them seem a play to the gallery. It was also the last time Rossouw came across as even remotely jocular. *2019-04-09*

What followed was the polar opposite of Noakes's presentation: a dry, measured delivery of a succession of slides showing graphs and reams of data designed to support his argument that cholesterol is an important risk factor for heart disease and that current dietary recommendations do more good than harm. It was acutely detailed and unapologetically academic. It was also a science journalist's nightmare. I was not surprised. Scientists find solace in data; streams of figures are their Linus's blanket; all commentary needs to be qualified and quantifiable. Journalists, however, feel more at ease with the creative licence allowed with words. It's why many scientists I know distrust the media. Rossouw was certainly not speaking with an unqualified audience in mind. It was as if he had a secret. Somewhere buried within the incessant flow of data and the squiggly lines on the graphs was a thread of thought, an argument, a narrative that I, and other non-specialists in the room, had to try to decode.

I shook my head and looked at my notebook. There were puzzled question marks everywhere, together with half-finished sentences, scribbles and words that would demand follow-up research. But my interest had been piqued.

The essence of his argument was familiar: that low-density lipoprotein (LDL, or 'bad') cholesterol build-up in the arteries was the consequence of eating saturated (largely animal) fats such as those found in dairy products and red meat, or trans (largely artificial) fats such as those found in cakes, pies and potato chips, and was the principal cause of the build-up of plaque in the arteries. This constricted blood flow and contributed to the development of CHD. As a consequence, people were better off minimising the intake of such fats.

I was interested to see how Noakes was going to reply; after all, this was supposed to be a debate – the Great Centenary Debate, remember? Both of them were to present an argument, the other was then allowed to reply or challenge, and then the event was to be opened up to the audience for questions. But the scheduled rebuttal of Rossouw's argument by Noakes never happened. Instead, the two were quickly seated side by side, Rossouw looking somewhat diminutive next to Noakes's lanky frame. They then faced the court of informed opinion. Noakes smiled, clearly expecting to be challenged but nonetheless a little thrown by this turn of events. Then, seemingly unperturbed, his mood confidently cavalier and his passion for the topic unshakeable, he started fielding the questions, and for a while he was on a roll, unstoppable. But then things changed. Something started chiselling away at his energy, and he seemed to grow tired, frustrated and anxious.

While the focus in the room continually shifted between the audience and the two panellists, I never took my eyes off Noakes; I could see how the constant barrage from those before him was starting to take its toll. He seemed to slump in his seat, his body bowed, that seemingly ever-present smile slipping from his face. I was relatively new to the customs of academic debate, but even I could sense that there was something uncharacteristically brutal in what was playing out. As if to add insult to injury, Rossouw was becoming emboldened by his opponent's public excoriation. He began peppering his comments and answers with subtle barbs, delivered with quiet relish.

As I watched Noakes, I wondered why he was doing this. A stream of questions started to instinctively find their way to my front of mind. I was a little out of my league covering sports science and human nutrition, but now Noakes was stumbling onto my 'patch': the complex interface of science, the media and human behaviour. The journalist in me immediately saw a story: why was this reserved man, a seasoned academic and a globally respected authority in his field, leading what seemed a quixotic charge against the established tenets of another branch of science? Was he mistaken, or had he stumbled across something? If so, ~2019-04-09~ what was driving him to risk injury to his reputation and endure accusations and comments that clearly hurt him?

I needed to know.

Chapter 2

'Newton, we have a problem': The uncomfortable truth about science and human nature

Before we get to know Tim Noakes better, we need some context. How you interpret what he says depends to a large degree on your relationship with science, and I'm willing to bet it's rather strained. That's not your fault. You're very much a victim of history, science and the media. We'll get to the last two later; first of all, we need to go back in time.

20190409

If I were to ask you to name an influential ancient Chinese philosopher, the chances are you'll say Confucius. Indeed, his name has become something of an epithet for wisdom. But ask philosophers of science, and they'll more than likely invoke the name of Mo Di, or, as he later became known, Mo Tzu (an honorific title meaning Master Mo). He was a celebrated Chinese

Good to explain.

philosopher active during the late 5th to the early 4th centuries BCE. He had studied Confucianism at school, but found its canonical dictates with their unquestioning devotion to rituals and a rigid social order restrictive. He branched off to develop a school of philosophy that encouraged the questioning of authority and a concern for the welfare of others. This became known as Mohism, and its influence spread throughout what is now Asia. Mo Di was also a firm proponent of peace between states. All this was much to the concern of dictatorial regimes that demanded unquestioning obedience, the entrenchment of privilege and a predilection for war to address any challenge. Mo Di also laid the foundations for the development of physics, maths and mechanics in ancient China.

But that's not why he's in this story. It was many years after his death that things really got interesting, with the rise to power of Qin Shi Huang, the first emperor of China (it was a self-appointed title). He is afforded his place in history as the man who sowed the seeds for the modern state we know as China; the name comes from the Qin dynasty he founded. He unified the country (until then a collection of warring states), and went about establishing the standardisation of practices and measurements throughout the nation. Of course this couldn't be done without widespread acts of force designed to ensure submission to his dictates. These included the marginalisation of any schools of thought that questioned his authority, Mohism being chief among them. In the 3rd century BCE, Qin oversaw the extensive burning of books devoted to Mohism and, reportedly, had any scholars who protested buried alive. The Chinese historian Sima Qian recorded all this.

It is one of the first documented suppressions of free thought and philosophy – the precursor to science – by a controlling authority. Since then science has sat rather uncomfortably with various authorities. It's at this point that it would be logical to invoke religion. However, religion has at times been a strange bedfellow in the growth of science. During part of the Middle Ages – between the 8th and 13th centuries BCE – there was, parallel to the spread of Islam, a dramatic growth in medieval Islamic science that built upon ancient Arab, Persian, Indian and

Greek learning. Some of the key foundations of modern science – experimentation, scientific enquiry and clinical trials – were born at this time, as were other major achievements in astronomy, medicine and mathematics; in fact, the terms algebra and algorithm are Arabic in origin. This so-called Islamic Golden Age also saw rapid developments in arts, culture, technology, agriculture, economics and law. If there were a geographic nexus of all this learning and exchange of ideas, it was the city of Baghdad; ironic and tragic, given its current state. Various reasons have been given for the collapse of the Islamic Golden Era, including invasions from the Mongol Empire to the East and the Crusades from the West, and the reactive rise of the more hard-line Sunni Islam, which gave more sway to the voice of religious leaders. No surprise there.

Of course, religion and science don't normally go hand in hand. During the 16th and 17th centuries, European philosophers and scientists who questioned the authority of the Catholic Church were considered heretics and ripe for incarceration, their books burnt or banned. Among the most famous were Nicolaus Copernicus and Galileo Galilei, who had the temerity to present proof that the Earth revolved around the Sun and not vice versa, as was carried in the Holy Scriptures (it was only in 1820 that the church grudgingly acceded that science was right on the matter).

Science fought back, though, and that period is characterised by a scientific revolution in Europe that stood shoulder to shoulder with its philosophical ally and gave birth to some of the more familiar names to modern scholars of Western philosophy and science: Gottfried Leibniz, Thomas Hobbes, Francis Bacon, René Descartes, Edmond Halley, Johannes Kepler, Blaise Pascal and, of course, Isaac Newton.

What is surprising is that none of these were really 'scientists', at least not at the time. During this period, what we today call

16

'science' was an extension of philosophy, so those who fused the questioning discipline of philosophy with the study of the natural world were called 'natural philosophers', or referred to by the ~~2019 0409~~ German word *naturforscher*, naturalist. There were terms for those who studied other, more specific disciplines – chemist, mathematician – but not for the overall, more systematic enterprise of science. The term 'scientist' only really came into being in the 19th century; in fact in 1834, when it first appeared in print in a review by the English philosopher William Whewell of a book by Mary Somerville, one of the few women to stab her heel into the almost exclusive male domain of 19th-century science. Whewell harrumphed that just as someone who immerses him- or herself in art is deemed an artist, perhaps someone who immerses him- or herself in science should be called a 'scientist'.

Over time Whewell seemed to grow quite pleased with his idea, and in 1840 published a book titled *The Philosophy of the Inductive Science*, in which he famously wrote the following: 'As we cannot use physician for a cultivator of physics, I have called him a physicist. We need very much a name to describe a cultivator of science in general. I should incline to call him a Scientist. Thus we might say, that as an Artist is a Musician, Painter, or Poet, a Scientist is a Mathematician, Physicist, or Naturalist.'

Why this is important is because by using the term 'scientist' as a counterpoint to the term 'artist', Whewell was acknowledging a period of intense tension at the time between science and the arts. The first half of the 19th century in Europe was characterised by a growth of Romanticism, when leading figures in art, literature, politics and the humanities were fighting against what they saw as the reductionism of science. According to Wolf Lepenies in his book *Between Literature and Science: The Rise of Sociology* (1985), belief at the time was 'that calculation and measurement might displace cultivation and compassion', and there was a 'presumed threat which secular knowledge of all kinds posed to religious belief and practical piety'.

William Blake, the poet and poster boy for English Romanticism, didn't mince his words in his condemnation of science: 'Art', he wrote, 'is The Tree of Life. Science is the Tree of Death.' This rejection of science as a mechanic, reducing everything to its constituent parts, didn't dissipate. D.H. Lawrence later anguished on behalf of his fellow writers and poets: 'The Universe is dead for us, and how is it to come alive again … now that "knowledge" has killed the sun, making it a ball of gas, with spots'. Champions of the communication of science, people like Carl Sagan and more lately Richard Dawkins, of course reject this notion and point to the magnificent marvels of the natural world that have been brought to light under the careful scrutiny of science. I urge you to read Sagan's *Billions and Billions* and Dawkins's *The Greatest Show on Earth*.

However, despite the work of people like Sagan and Dawkins, the tension between what could be called 'the arts' and 'science' still exists. Part of this is the result of an inherited education system that for centuries favoured the humanities over science. It's easy to think that what we know as science stood alongside the humanities in some of the world's greatest universities, but that was not the case. In the UK, for example (whose education system South Africa inherited), according to Stefan Collini, science was considered 'a vocational and slightly grubby activity, not altogether suitable for the proper education of a gentleman'. Collini wrote this in his introduction to a seminal publication that emerged from an event that captured this tension. It was a lecture at Cambridge University on 7 May 1959 by a novelist called Charles Percy Snow, and his story warrants telling.

Snow was an early 20th-century British chemist who specialised in infrared spectroscopy. In 1932 he published a paper in *Nature* – one of science's most respected journals – claiming that vitamin A could be produced through artificial methods. As vitamin A deficiency was a major problem in poor countries, this was an exciting development in science; or so it was thought, until it emerged that his calculations were a little off track. The paper was withdrawn, and the reaction from the scientific community was brutal. Snow responded by abandoning scientific research to become a successful writer, lecturer and social commentator. He was so respected in these endeavours that he was awarded 20 honorary degrees and eventually received a peerage – he became Baron Snow in 1964. However, he never lost his deep respect for science.

When he was asked by his alma mater, Cambridge, to present the prestigious annual Rede Lecture in May 1959, expectation was that he would discuss his literary work. Instead, he presented a talk that would reverberate around academia worldwide. It was titled 'The Two Cultures and the Scientific Revolution'. The 'two cultures' were those of the grounded natural scientists and the more effete 'literary intellectuals'. He felt qualified to speak about both cultures because, in his words, 'by training I was a scientist: by vocation I was a writer'. Importantly, Snow claimed that between the cultures was 'a profound mutual suspicion and incomprehension', which in turn was hindering the application of technology to global problems. He was quite unrestrained (for an academic): 'The non-scientists have a rooted impression that the scientists are shallowly optimistic, unaware of man's condition. On the other hand, the scientists believe that the literary intellectuals are totally lacking in foresight, particularly unconcerned with their brother man.' But when it came to the crunch, Snow showed a gravity towards those for whom the disciplined examination of the natural world held the most acclaim, and who, ironically, many years previous had been unremitting in his opprobrium: 'In the moral, they are by and large the soundest group of intellectuals we have; there is a moral component right in the grain of science itself, and almost all scientists form their own judgement of the moral life.'

When reviews of 'The Two Cultures', both the lecture and the book that followed, were published, the condemnation, especially by literary commentators who saw Snow as a turncoat, was brutal. Importantly, however, there was little challenge to Snow's overall premise of a deleterious tension between the humanities and science, especially within the realms of tertiary education.

Has that tension been tempered over the years? I'd argue that in its wake, there is still the enduring perception that the two – science and the arts – somehow exist as separate conceptual applications. Indeed, the belief that the brain has two hemispheres – a left that is more analytical and a right that is more creative – pervades, even though there is increasing evidence that this is not the case and that both hemispheres are actually intricately connected in their conceptual processing. And yet this conceptual bifurcation has been used as the basis for dividing children's educational paths – especially at Western schools – as either towards the arts or towards the sciences; even more incredulously in the bizarre gender stereotyping that boys are better at the sciences, girls the arts.

What is more pervasive is an almost conceptual ring-fencing of science as something that scientists *do*, as opposed to something that unlocks our understanding of every single part of our natural world – both that outside us and within us. There seems to be an almost sapient-centric arrogance that humans are of principal importance, and that very little else needs to be considered beyond that which supports our immediate cause. If there is any deference, it is to an imaginary god or gods, rather than the contextual realisation that in the greater, natural scheme of things, humans are not that important. Douglas Adams says it best in the immortal opening lines of *The Hitchhiker's Guide to the Galaxy*: 'Far out in the uncharted backwaters of the unfashionable end of the Western Spiral arm of the Galaxy lies a small unregarded yellow sun. Orbiting this at a distance of roughly ninety-eight million miles is an utterly insignificant little blue-green planet whose ape-descended life forms are so amazingly primitive that they still think digital watches are a pretty neat idea.'

This questioning of authority as championed by Mo Tzu thousands of years ago is a cornerstone of science. In the words of noted astrophysicist Neil deGrasse Tyson, as host of the recent adaptation of Carl Sagan's epic TV series *Cosmos*, 'Science needs the light of free expression to flourish; it needs the fearless questioning of authority and the open exchange of ideas.' Whereas science has no Vatican, no central authority, there is something akin to its spiritual home: the Royal Society, the UK's national science academy. Its motto, *Nullius in verba* (meaning 'Take nobody's word for it'), is an unequivocal call to question everything without fear or favour. And that means *it* is feared, by authorities around the world, be they governments, large corporations, cultural organisations or, of course, religious institutions, who see the advancement of scientific knowledge as a challenge to their status quo, or, more specifically, that science is 'playing God'.

Contraception is a case in point. Even in the face of the scourge of HIV/AIDS, and more recently the Zika virus, the Catholic Church has remained steadfast that contraception is an abomination, or as parodied by the Monty Python team in *The Meaning of Life*, every sperm is sacred. Mary Stopes, commenting on the inevitable clerical objections to contraception, recalled the criticism at the time towards inoculation against smallpox: '[it] was denounced as being "indefensible on religious as well as medical grounds"…"a diabolical operation"…"a discovery sent into the world by the powers of evil"'. Science eradicated smallpox; until a vaccination is found for HIV/AIDS, the dithering of the church around contraception threatens the lives of millions of Catholics.

Religion is possibly the single biggest destructive force in the shaping of public opinion towards science, and the chances are that it's not going to go away any time soon. The eminent American biologist Edward O. Wilson, in his influential treatise *On Human Nature*, says that 'the predisposition to religious belief is the most complex and powerful force in the human mind and, in all probability an ineradicable part of human nature'. He points to the discoveries of bone altars and displays of funeral rites in Neanderthal dwellings as evidence that the belief in spirits may go back as far as over 60 000 years, and references Canadian-American anthropologist Anthony F.C. Wallace, who said that since then mankind has produced about 100 000 religions.

That there have been so many different religions, of course, would be dismissed by those who think theirs is unique and therefore somehow incontrovertible. In *God Is Not Great*, Christopher Hitchens reminds those who anchor their faith in the distinctive tale of a virgin or miraculous birth that human belief has been there before: the Greek demigod Perseus was apparently born when the god Jupiter visited the virgin Danaë as a shower of gold that made her pregnant; the god Buddha was born through the opening in his mother's flank; Genghis Khan was reportedly born of the virgin daughter of a Mongol king after she awoke one night and found herself bathed in a great light; the Hindu god Krishna was born of the virgin Devaka; the Egyptian god Horus was born of the goddess Isis (but only after she had retrieved all the dismembered body parts of her murdered husband Osiris, except his penis, which was eaten by catfish); the Roman god Mercury was born of the virgin Maia; and the ancient Phrygo-

Roman god Attis is often depicted as being born of a virgin mother on, wait for it, December 25th.

Despite all the corroboration that the current dominant religions are essentially mishmashes of belief systems that have existed over thousands of years; that they imaginatively and creatively metamorphosed through word-of-mouth retellings until they were seized upon by powerful institutions that crafted them for their own purposes; that they are open to all manner of interpretations; and that each religion has a myriad offshoots, each of which stakes a claim to authenticity, often delivered with unremitting bloodletting, adherents of a religion will unquestioningly reject the clear evidence of science and fill its place with an amalgam of cherry-picked wild tales. And yet those same people will gladly embrace all the benefits that science provides, such as medicine and technology.

2019-04-09

This points to a very powerful cognitive dissonance that attempts to balance some of the fundamental differences between religion and science. One of those is that whereas religion invokes a fictional supreme authority that must be obeyed, science fearlessly questions not only authority, but also itself.

Carl Sagan develops this thought in *Billions and Billions*, the last book that he wrote before he died, by explaining how the methods and ethos of religion and science are profoundly different: 'Religion frequently asks us to believe without question, even (or especially) in the absence of hard evidence. Indeed, this is the central meaning of faith. Science asks us to take nothing on faith, to be wary of our penchant for self-deception, to reject anecdotal evidence. Science considers deep skepticism a prime virtue. Religion often sees it as a barrier to enlightenment. So, for centuries, there has been a conflict between the two fields – the discoveries of science challenging religious dogmas, and religion attempting to ignore or suppress the disquieting findings.'

2019-04-09

And whereas the one generates regressive conflict, the other creates intellectual growth. Bill Nye, in his book *Undeniable: Evolution and the Science of Creation*, explains it thus: 'When religions disagree about just creation, there is nothing to do but argue. When two scientists disagree about evolution, they confer with colleagues, develop theories, collect evidence, and arrive at a more complete understanding. Every question leads to new answers, new discoveries, and new smarter questions.'

The result of modern scientific knowledge competing with religions forged in antiquity is a society with a rather uncomfortable relationship with science. People will accept the science behind a cellphone, but say the science that shows humans and apes evolved from a common ancestor must be flawed. They may even accept that the church was wrong about the Earth being the centre of the universe, but that it's still spot on with the assertion that the Earth is only 6 000 years old.

How is it possible then that religion and science still coexist? The answer could lie, ironically, within science. Kevin Nelson, a leading neurologist at the University of Kentucky and one of the world's most renowned authorities on near-death experiences, believes religion could be 'hot-wired' into our brains. According to his book *The God Impulse*, 'Our spiritual experiences have instinctual qualities, originating in the most primitive parts of our brains ... They appear intertwined with the brain's limbic structures, which produce feelings and emotions.' Essentially he says that what we interpret as the spiritual experiences that are requisite for an emotional connection with religion are little more than instinctive activity in the brain. As an example, he explains that the 'light at the end of a tunnel' experience of people at near death, which is consequently interpreted as the calling of heaven, is nothing more than the result of not enough blood being pumped to the head, causing the eyes' blood vessels to constrict

and choke off blood supply, resulting in the loss of peripheral 2019·04·09
vision. There is nothing 'heavenly' about it; it's basic human
physiology, the body being the body, and humans with insuffi-
cient scientific knowledge making up stories to try to explain it.

Another leading researcher in the search for physical sources
of spiritual consciousness is Michael Persinger, a neuropsycholo-
gist at Canada's Laurentian University in Ontario. Since the 1980s 2019·04·09
he has been electrically stimulating parts of the brains of conscious subjects and discovered that when certain separate parts
of the brain, believed to be normally responsible for developing
a sense of 'self', are stimulated at the same time, the resultant
'short-circuiting' elicits a sensation of the shadowy presence of
another entity. The context of each subject's upbringing rushes
in to attach meaning to this 'sensed presence'; it becomes, for
example, Mohammed, the Virgin Mary, the Sky Spirit, or a long-
dead family member. It must be pointed out that Persinger's work
is controversial, but that doesn't mean it shouldn't be considered.

We are not born distrustful of science, we are taught it. Like
racism, homophobia or any other prejudice, it is the outcome
of the opinions – or ignorance – of parents, teachers and communities, and the complicity of religion in this regard cannot be
overemphasised. The shaping of attitudes towards science is not
limited to the community-level preaching in churches, temples
and mosques, or the propaganda taught in the schools they 2019·04·09
control; it's in their continued influence at state level. This can
be overt, as in the control of Iran's Islamic theologians over the
election of their Supreme Leader, the deceptively quaint symbiosis between the British monarchy and the Anglican Church, or
the more dissembling claims of separation of church and state
in the US, while the command 'In God we trust' still holds court in
their legislative chambers and courtrooms. Or it can be covert –
on a subtler level, acquiescence to the dictates of religions lies in

the national celebration of religious holidays and the invocation of deities in national anthems, South Africa's *Nkosi Sikelel' iAfrika* being a case in point.

20190409   Yet, science is the only way of accurately understanding our natural world; anything else is make-believe. The unequivocal proof thereof is in the replicable application of science: technology. So much of what we take for granted as part of our modern world has been realised only by using science to understand – and thoroughly test – the underlying hypotheses. Bolts of lightning, formerly considered portents of doom or the designs of sorcerers, can be recreated in a laboratory. Heavier-than-air craft take to the skies daily because of our clear understanding of pressure differentials produced by the shape of a bird's wing, not because those aboard all pray to the powers of an omnipotent being. Despite Christian Scientists believing that a child's fever, headaches and stiffness of the neck emanate from that child's impure thoughts, modern medicine's understanding of germ theory, and the technology it has produced, means we can do a simple test for meningitis, and if that is proved the case, treat the child with antibiotics. Of course the parents would probably disagree, refuse medication in accordance with their beliefs, and let the child die in excruciating pain while they stand beside his or her bed, their heads bowed in deference to the imaginary. In his book *The Demon-Haunted World*, Carl Sagan explains this with typical eloquence: 'Microbiology and meteorology now explain what only a few centuries ago was considered sufficient cause to burn women to death.'

And that's what frustrates scientists. Popular superstitions, religious beliefs and the mistrust of science still abound, despite all the evidence from science that we happily embrace in medicine and technology. A lot of it has to do with defects in human nature, specifically how we cheat and deceive at cognition.

From the moment we are born, we try to make sense of the world around us. Signals from our five senses – touch, taste, sight, smell and hearing – are transmitted to our brain, and for the purposes of instinctive self-preservation are processed and catalogued. Our early ancestors would have learnt that the rustle of grass meant the possible presence of not only prey, but also of a predator, and therefore demanded extra vigilance. The smell of carrion – manna from heaven for hyenas – is offensive to humans because we don't have the gastric mechanism for filtering out the dangerous pathogens that accompany decaying meat. We know this now because research shows that carrion-eaters generally have a lower pH (higher acidity) level in their stomachs. Our ancestors would have learnt this the hard way, however, and then passed on this knowledge until it became genetically imprinted into our DNA as a gagging reflex.

But the human brain, considered the most evolved compared to those of all our fellow mammals, is not averse to being lazy. In fact, it's key for the brain's survival. If the brain were to continually process the raw data input purely from our eyes as *new* data, in real time, it would likely overheat. Instead, the path between visual input and perception is an intricate weave of conscious and unconscious visual snapshots and cognitive assumptions gathered over time. The result is a continual time-averaged composite of the immediate and the past; it's as if the eyes 'see' dots and the brain joins them together – based on previous experiences – in order to make sense of them. According to Jason Fischer, a neuroscientist at the Massachusetts Institute of Technology and author of a research paper titled 'Serial dependence in visual perception': 'What you are seeing at the present moment is not a fresh snapshot of the world but rather an average of what you've seen in the past 10 to 15 seconds.' This is why the brain is so easily fooled; illusionists and tricksters depend on it.

One of the ways the brain takes a short cut in processing information is in the constructing of, especially familiar, patterns and the allocating of signals to those patterns. This is why a random cloud can take on the shape of a chicken or the wind through the trees can sound like someone breathing heavily. This simplification process – the attempt by the brain to pigeonhole something new into our cognitive construct – has a term: pareidolia. Notch this up a bit, and these patterns take on meaning: burn marks on a piece of toast look like the Virgin Mary, or the voice in a recording played backwards tells you the aliens are coming. This perception of connections and *meaningfulness* of unrelated phenomena is called apophenia. In each case there's a clear scientific explanation for what is being experienced through our senses, but the human brain is suggesting otherwise. The key to seeing beyond the familiar patterns to what is really happening is critical thinking, and it is the 'critical' component to thinking that is, well, critical, because without it, we're suckers for snake oil or, to use a more modern term, pseudoscience.

Here's a quick test. Which of the following is a recognised branch of science?: astrology, telepathy, dianetics, three-cycle biorhythms, precognition, numerology, phrenology, telekinesis, homeopathy. It is, of course, a trick question. They are all forms of pseudoscience; as such they present themselves as consistent with all the conventions of scientific research (complete with impressive, sciencey-sounding names), but in fact fail miserably when confronted with the rigours of qualified scientific enquiry.

So how is it possible that even people living in developed countries, with a good-quality education and who have been exposed to the joys of science, believe in such highly illogical and scientifically unproven rubbish as astrology, numerology and homeopathy? There are several reasons (and these may sound a little familiar): because it is part of their culture, an ancestral 'wisdom' passed down over hundreds of years through various forms, including word of mouth by so-called leaders; and because part of that same culture is to not question the authority of these leaders.

Many of these pseudoscientific lines of thought have their roots in pre-scientific thinking, but have remained in our culture because they are attractive and can be used to weave wonderful stories that capture our imagination ('you're going to meet a tall, dark and handsome stranger'). But because they are non-scientific, and therefore malleable, these ancient beliefs can also be shaped and wielded by charlatans, who then use them to lead people in dangerous directions.

What about the new pseudoscience that continually works its way into our world? What about the laughable fads like 'The Secret' or the more sinister movements like Intelligent Design? Why is it that seemingly rational people get drawn into their vortex like birds sucked into an aeroplane engine? Because people don't examine what's before them, and, despite being blessed with an incredibly developed brain, they don't think critically. They believe, unquestioningly, anything that's dressed up like science, and they are attracted to confident and charismatic people who tell them that something works. That's why critical thinking is the difference between thinking someone's a prophet and knowing they're a charlatan.

There's another reason why pseudoscience exists: science doesn't know everything. If it did, in the words of my favourite comedian and fellow sceptic Dara Ó Briain, it would stop. Pseudoscience continually points to the absence of knowledge as an invitation to be creative with the truth. It's a little like finding a dropped pen at a crime scene and accordingly arresting any accountant selected randomly from the phone book.

Carl Sagan wrote in *The Demon-Haunted World*, 'Scientists are used to struggling with Nature, who may surrender her secrets

reluctantly but who fights fair.' What he means is that in the vast-
ness of the natural world, there's still a lot we don't know, but if
we examine it methodically and, importantly, critically, we will
get to understand it; however, if we cut corners or misrepresent
it, we will pay dearly.

The result of this failure in science to rush in and answer
fundamental questions about the world around us has left a lot
still to be discovered. And that's exciting. But it has a downside.
If the scope of scientific enquiry – from quarks to quasars and
everything around and in between – was an ocean, what we currently know would only be a single, albeit wonderfully equipped,
lifeboat, and pseudoscience would be the flotsam that desperate,
unthinking people cling to. It would be brightly coloured but
dangerous flotsam with hidden sharp edges, and unfortunately
there'd be a lot of it.

We would all like to think that we are beyond being fooled by
pseudoscience. That we are rational creatures, that the opinions
and decisions we make are based on evidence and clear thinking. We would probably acquiesce that, yes, every now and then
we may make a decision based on an emotional reaction, and
acknowledge that our subconscious thoughts might, occasionally,
bubble to the surface, but in general we're pretty level-headed.
The reality may be a little more frightening. In his book *Heretics:
Adventures with the Enemies of Science*, the journalist Will Storr
meets a stream of people typically derided by sceptics, including
homoeopaths, past-life regression therapists and UFO spotters,
and is intrigued by how they fiercely adhere to their beliefs even
though the scientific establishment has long since debunked
them. It seems that they only see what they want to see, and
ignore what they don't; they seem to edit their memories to their
advantage; and, importantly, when challenged, their instinct seems
to hold more fiercely to their beliefs. And it's not just them, says

Storr, it's everyone. He describes the human brain as 'an organ of bias and prejudice whose rapid responses are made possible by its models – stubborn approximations of how the world works'.

That does not mean there isn't a little wiggle room. According to American neuroscientist and writer David Eagleman of Stanford University and the Center for Science and Law, the mind is not a single thinking-centre, but a combination of 'sub-agents' with different agendas. In his book *Incognito: The Secret Lives of the Brain*, he describes the mind as built of overlapping 'experts' that weigh in and compete over different choices, and who are locked in chronic battle. Your behaviour, according to Eagleman, 'is simply the end result of the battles'. Unfortunately, the unconscious and emotional 'experts' are heavily armed and highly persuasive.

All this would suggest that if you think carefully and critically, aware that what you see and hear may not be what is real, then perhaps, just perhaps, you'd be able to know the truth about the world around you through the discipline of science.

Unfortunately, science is not everything it's cracked up to be.

Is this chapter for Noakes or against? Or neutral? 2019-04-09

Chapter 3

When science drops the ball: The uncomfortable truth about the nature of science

Scientific knowledge comes with caveats: it is at best incomplete, at worst wrong, most likely somewhere in between. At issue is the scope and complexity of the subject matter (our natural world); the robustness demanded of the way we examine it (the scientific method); the demands, frailties and idiosyncrasies of those implementing it (the scientists); and the resultant disconnects, which are euphemistically referred to as 'dodgy science'.

Let's dig deeper into the issue of complexity. If you ever find yourself with a little time on your hands, I urge you to look up a paper titled 'Alternative reproductive tactics and male-dimorphism in the horned beetle *Onthophagus acuminatus*' by Douglas J. Emlen, an evolutionary biologist and Professor of Biology at the University of Montana in the US. It's a fascinating and entertaining paper about the males of this particular species of dung beetle – which have a pair of horns that protrude from the base of the head – and how their reproductive behaviour differs according to the size of their horns. Those with more intimidating horns guard tunnels leading to the females, while those with smaller horns find devious ways of reaching them – the females, not the tunnels – such as digging new tunnels that intercept those guarded by the males with the really big horns.

Now let's put Professor Emlen's paper into context: it's just one paper that touches on one specific form of behaviour of just one of approximately 2000 species that form part of the genus *Onthophagus* (from the Greek for dung eater), which is part of the family Scarabaeidae (or scarab beetles), of which there are about 30 000 species in total, which makes up a fraction of a larger family, Scarabaeoidea, which is only one part of the order Coleoptera (all beetles), which is part of the larger class Insecta (all insects, of which there are well over 900 000 species), which is just one of many phyla that include other invertebrates such as crabs and spiders, which are part of the larger animal kingdom (that includes mammals, such as us humans), which is one of five kingdoms of living things on our planet (the others are plants, fungi, monera – such as bacteria – and protists – such as algae).

And that's just living things. There are also scientists like Emlen examining every single component – from the invisible to the microscopic to the visible – of the *inanimate* world in which we live, including everything to do with the air around it, the immediate space around that world, all the known components in the solar system in which our planet resides, every known component of the billions of stars in our galaxy, and every one of the billion known galaxies in our known universe. Oh yes, and there are theoretical physicists who study what is believed to be the myriad multiverses, of which our universe is just one. And then there are those who examine the chemical building blocks of all of that, and those who delve even deeper into the subatomic building blocks of those building blocks.

I have probably left out other disciplines, and for that I apologise, but I think you get the point. And here's the kicker: for every paper like Emlen's that is published, there are other scientists who *must* challenge it, because science is driven by that motto of the Royal Society: *nullius in verba* – take nobody's word for it.

There have been many attempts to explain what science is – that it's a discipline, an authority, a method, a body of knowledge, a human endeavour; and, yes, it's all of those, but I think that just confuses the matter. So I'm going to suggest another descriptive tag that embraces all of this, that captures its complexity and the role that humans play in it, and it's one I suspect many scientists won't like, but here it is anyway: science is a game. It's an ongoing tussle between humans in all their idiosyncratic fallibility and Nature in all her beguiling perfection.

This game of science has players and, importantly, it has rules. And Nature may fight fair, but she's reluctant to surrender her secrets. She is continually adapting to everything we throw at her, and the resultant complexity of the game means that humans have to be both creative in our strategy and methodical in our tactics if we are to gain even a foothold.

To make things even more complex, there is no single strategy for scientists to keep their eye on the ball. Broadly speaking, there are two: one is epistemic, the other practical. These are sometimes referred to as the 'pure' or 'applied' sciences. The first focuses on the more academic pursuit of knowledge for knowledge's sake, whereas the latter focuses on the *application* of what is learnt to secure solutions to, essentially human, problems.

In my experience, having interviewed scientists across the spectrum of research, those involved in 'pure' research have a tendency to scoff at those in the applied sciences, who in turn dismiss the 'purists' as being out of touch with the demands of the real world. However, the idea that scientific research is more of a spectrum of application makes sense when you realise that if there is something that scientists engaging in both strategies search for, it is the 'truth' about our natural world. For those driven by more epistemic priorities, it's about the *integrity* or *purity* of the knowledge; for those with their eye on technical applications, the success (or failure) of those applications relies on the *accuracy* and *replicability* of that knowledge. Human nutrition is one of those branches of science that benefits from both pure and applied research.

In the search for 'truth', science needs to be both methodical and ethical. Unfortunately, both pursuits are marred by profound errors. The broadly speaking 'scientific method' is the methodological foundation for scientific research. It demands observation by a suitably qualified researcher of the natural world, the establishment of a hypothesis, the prediction of an outcome based on the hypothesis, the testing of that hypothesis through rigorous experimentation, and the submission of the outcomes, together with a conclusion, for peer review, where every component is checked, and re-checked, and if deemed rigorous enough, is published, where, theoretically, it encourages others to replicate the outcomes. If replication – with the same outcomes – is achieved, then it is considered part of that corpus of knowledge deemed approximate to the 'truth', something termed 'scientific consensus'. However, even then there's a seemingly paradoxical caveat: at any time, that considered 'truth' could be overturned by the advancement of the very science that says it is so. Case in point: Newton's clockwork theory, long considered the most accurate understanding of the universe, was upended by Einstein's theory that space and time are, in fact, relative.

To try to explain the seeming impermanence of scientific knowledge, science speaks of 'theories', but a scientific theory is not just an idea, some kind of thumb-suck wrapped in impressive and inaccessible (to most) mathematical notation. It is the closest we have to the complete understanding of a concept in

that

2019 0409

science, at that time, because all the evidence, usually across *multiple disciplines* within science, gives us the same conclusion. This means that a scientific theory – such as evolution by natural selection – as an in-depth explanation of a natural phenomenon (in this case the origins and diversity of all life) is usually embraced by most scientists. Having said that, it hasn't stopped some of the world's greatest minds – including Richard Dawkins in a book called *This Idea Must Die*, edited by John Brockman – from presenting their suggestions of theories that they believe are blocking the progress of science. Among them is the scientific method itself!

I hope at this stage you're not about to throw your arms up in exasperation, abandon your conviction in the clarity of science and embrace the ridiculousness of pseudoscience. My point here is to underpin a key component of the virtuousness of science: *its constant self-examination and disposition for adjustment in the face of new evidence.* And if you've got that, as I'm sure you have, you're going to need it, because your trust in science is about to be severely tested. The scientific method, albeit noble and disciplined, has inherent weaknesses, and these are especially evident when putting humans under the microscope.

Humans generally make bad subjects for research because they are hampered by the vagaries of human behaviour, all of which can introduce bias into a trial: they lie, they have prejudices, they yearn for social acceptance, they are susceptible to peer pressure, they are inclined to acquiesce to authority, and they are quick to embrace a simple answer over the burden of employing critical thinking. Oh yes, and biologically speaking, humans are quite possibly the most intricate animals on the planet, although I know one or two politicians that are clear exceptions.

The so-called gold standard of evidence collection – the randomised controlled trial – demands that when doing any manner of research that involves an intervention on humans (such as a

36

therapy, a form of medication or a change in diet), the following checks need to be in place: the subjects must be examined under clinical conditions where all possible extraneous variables are eliminated or mitigated to acceptable levels; the subjects should be *randomly* divided into at least two groups, one of which is a control group that receives no *active* intervention; and there must be clearly and carefully defined outcomes that are measurable. Ideally the trial should also be double-blind, meaning those applying the intervention have no idea if what they're applying is active or not. I can imagine you're already seeing problems when it comes to such research into human nutrition.

If we feed the feral fallibility of human nature into the exacting demands of scientific evidence collection, all sorts of problems come tumbling out. Firstly, any human subjects in a trial know they're in a trial and are therefore inclined to adapt their behaviour in some way. This is especially the case if the trial requires their verbal, or even non-verbal, responses to enquiry. Here they are prone to appealing to authority and what they sense is expected of them. Humans will be flexible with the truth if they're being judged.

All this means that researching humans can be very testing for scientists. But it can also be very valuable, because humans are the biggest beneficiaries of the applications of pure research. Think medicine, technology, food and the thousands of consumer products we use. There are many rewards for scientists who succeed in tapping into this. These include prestige, prizes, funding, even fame. So the temptation to sidestep the stumbling blocks of human complexity in research is ever-present.

There's a cartoon doing the rounds on the internet that seems to have tapped into the resultant agonies within the current research zeitgeist. It shows a white-bearded, bespectacled 19th-century scientist alongside a slick, smooth-shaven 21st-century scientist (they're both males, I note). The 19th-century scientist is thinking, 'I must find the explanation for this phenomenon in order to truly understand Nature.' In contrast, the 21st-century scientist is thinking, 'I must get the result that fits my narrative so I can get my paper into Nature' (*Nature* being the pre-eminent science journal).

This is an area of science that is of particular interest to Professor David Resnick, a leading bioethicist with a particular penchant for the ethics of scientific research, and it's important to have people like him keeping an eye on science. In his book *The Ethics of Science: An Introduction*, he devotes a significant amount of time to a core component to the veracity of science – the peer-review system.

Essentially the system works like this: a researcher submits a paper to a journal, normally one serving their field of research. The journal's editor will make an initial judgement as to whether it is worthy of further review. If it is, it is sent to experts in the field, who are referred to as referees or reviewers. They may or may not be on the board of the journal, but, importantly, they should not receive any payment for reviewing the paper; the recognition that comes with being considered a reviewer should be enough, although it should be pointed out that usually the authors of a paper do not know who the reviewers are. It's also important to remember that reviewers are themselves leading academics with the associated demands and workloads. Their responsibility, ideally, is to identify any faults in methodology, any inaccuracies in the interpretation of the data, and/or any ethical line-crossing.

After a paper is reviewed, the reviewers decide whether or not to publish the paper, and, if yes, whether it should be published as is, or with minor or major revisions – the more the revisions, the more concerns the reviewers have with the exactness of the paper's contents or construction. Once published, it is considered worthy of inviting professional challenges from other scientists; and challenge they do. They submit suggestions of where errors were made, and provide evidence from other research to back themselves up. If a paper is online, this can be done immediately. Authors of papers can then publish clarifications, corrections or even retractions to address any problems that are identified.

Resnick explains that the system functions as a quality-control mechanism by distinguishing between high- and low-quality research papers submitted to journals, and how the editors of those journals (supposedly) only publish papers of high quality. 2019-04-09 Papers are judged on various standards of argumentation and evidence, methodology and writing. Theoretically, this legitimises scientific knowledge. It also, supposedly, encourages honesty and objectivity, and eradicates any biases or errors that may have crept into the methodology.

The cautious tone of my explanation so far should highlight the opportunities in the system for mistakes or sleight of hand; and there's plenty of evidence of that. For the same reason that 2019-04-09 humans make bad subjects for research, they're fallible mechanisms for reviewing. They are prone to bias, bad judgement and making mistakes. This means there's always the possibility that bad science can slip through the system's filters and find its way into the public realm.

There's also the issue of replicability. Any experimental find- 2019-04-09 ing published in a journal should, ideally, be replicated by other scientists to test its outcomes. However, the human nature of scientists encourages them to pursue novel research with their eyes on all the sparkly prizes mentioned earlier. This means that a lot 2019-04-09 of previous research is not replicated and is therefore untested. This is one of the issues presented by John Ioannidis, Professor of Medicine, of Health Research and Policy, and of Statistics at

Stanford University, in a landmark paper published in 2005, titled, rather unambiguously, 'Why most published research findings are false'. He says, 'Several methodologists have pointed out that the high rate of non-replication (lack of confirmation) of research discoveries is a consequence of the convenient, yet ill-founded strategy of claiming conclusive research findings solely on the basis of a single study.' This is dangerous for the advancement of science, which normally doesn't manifest itself in dramatic leaps, but rather in small, tentative steps that are continually tested before reaching any measure of scientific consensus.

There's another, more insidious, problem with the peer-review system, and again, it is one that bothers Ioannidis. It centres on an oft-forgotten fact about scientific research: the information that emerges is an economic commodity, and journals are a key medium of exchange of this commodity.

This is especially important when it comes to biomedical research, which focuses on the prevention and treatment of diseases that cause illness and death in humans. That image you may have of a biomedical scientist at a research hospital – hunched over a lab table in their clinically white lab coat, punching data into a computer, pausing every now and then to examine the contents of a conical flask, then calmly tottering off to a research conference to discuss their findings – is a little oversimplified. The harsh reality is that academics are under constant, tremendous pressure, and this is especially the case within any field of research continually expected to find solutions to human problems. And if there are two words that make many a biomedical researcher sob and extend a shaking hand to a flagon of wine, they are 'funding' and 'publish', and the two are tied to each other.

In September 2016 the Royal Society published a paper engagingly titled 'The natural selection of bad science'. Its authors – Paul E. Smaldino, Associate Professor in the Department of

Cognitive and Information Sciences at the Merced campus of the University of California, and Richard McElreath, director of the Department of Human Behavior, Ecology and Culture at the Max Planck Institute for Evolutionary Anthropology in Leipzig, Germany – hit the proverbial nail on the head: journal publication is a principal factor in a researcher's career advancement. Two components to publication are emphasised: the number of publications a researcher has under their belt, and the number of times any one of their publications is cited by another publication, something called impact factor. You don't have to be an academic to acknowledge that in the rush to publish, serious errors of judgement, bad research, faked results and simple mistakes are bound to take a hold.

Unfortunately, because scientific research drives innovation in fields such as medicine, pharmaceuticals, armaments, technology, agriculture, sport and nutrition, it can provide significant financial and political leverage. It has therefore attracted more than its fair share of villains: scientists misrepresenting their findings to fall in line with the demands of their sponsors; research organisations colouring their work to capture the imagination of an unsuspecting media; so-called alternative healing practitioners dressing up their 'therapies' in the guise of medicine; politicians twisting data to drive their agendas; lobby groups cherry-picking data to seemingly justify their cause; pharmaceutical companies suppressing research that exposes faults in their products; food supplement companies marketing products as critical components of a 'healthy lifestyle'; cosmetics companies lying about the toxicity of their products; and food and beverage multinationals peddling products with marginal, if any, nutritional value as 'part of a healthy, balanced meal'.

Nonetheless, within this mash of shoddy research, marketing spin, misrepresentation and downright criminal behaviour, science somehow manages to retain an element of structured integrity. The result is a developing assembly of authoritative knowledge with which the bulk of scientists agree. This then becomes what is referred to as evidence-based, conventional scientific knowledge.

But then, every now and then, a scientist comes along, takes that conventional wisdom by the scruff of the neck and gives it a good shake. They do so for any one of a number of reasons: an acrimonious disregard for authority; an overly cavalier approach to their work; a larger-than-life lifestyle and public image; or because they have unearthed something that others had missed. For their effrontery to the conformities of the discipline, they pay the price. They are often pilloried, shunned, publicly ridiculed, even excommunicated; and yet they are essential to the very health of science. They encourage it to re-examine conventional wisdom and, where necessary, prune it; occasionally even uproot it. They are the mavericks; sometimes they're good for science, sometimes they're bad.

Most people familiar with the term 'maverick' would consider it negative, reserved for someone who doesn't toe the line, or who upsets the balance of things, often at the expense of others. This is inaccurate, and unfortunate. The *Oxford English Dictionary* has two explanations for 'maverick': the first being an 'unorthodox or independent-minded person', and the second 'an unbranded calf or yearling'. The connection between the two has an interesting story, and can be traced back to 19th-century America, the birth of a state, and a brave man who didn't want to hurt his cows.

His name was Samuel Augustus Maverick, and he was a highly successful 19th-century Texan lawyer, land baron, businessman and politician, and a central figure in the lead up to, and signing of, the Texas Declaration of Independence. He was also an incidental and somewhat reluctant cattle breeder, after receiving

42

a herd of cattle as part payment for outstanding rental. Partly because of his relative disinterest in ranching, and partly out of concern for the welfare of the cows, he refused to have the cattle branded, and let them wander across his land. This was counter to common practice. Neighbouring farmers took to labelling such wandering, unbranded cattle as 'mavericks', and were sometimes not averse to absorbing them into their own herds.

It's fair to say that Samuel Maverick was not as successful in cattle ranching as he was in his other business pursuits. By most accounts, though, he was considered by many of his personal friends as unconventional, free-thinking and patriotic; and therefore possibly best suited to developing the legislative framework for a fledgling state. For this reason, he holds a special place as something of a hero in the history of the state of Texas.

However, his most lasting legacy is the adoption of his name into the English language to describe someone who is unconventional, unorthodox or dissident, and who, in the process, sometimes sets new trends.

Science has seen its fair share of mavericks. Of the 'good' mavericks, there are those who immediately spring to mind, not only because their impact on science was profound, but also because it was not before they endured their fair share of rebuke from friends and colleagues. The best known is Albert Einstein.

Prior to the early 20th century, Sir Isaac Newton was the dominant force in our understanding of physics, especially gravity. In Newton's universe, masses exerted a force on each other and space existed independent of the celestial bodies within it. Importantly, both space and time were absolute. Einstein unwound Newton's so-called clockwork universe and replaced it with one where everything was relative, where clocks could run slower or faster, theoretically even backwards, depending on the speed of travel through, or relative position within, the universe. According to Einstein, space and time were neither separate nor absolute, but woven together into a single fabric he called 'spacetime'. Needless to say, his theory was initially rejected by a science community very comfortable with the way things were. Sceptics pointed to his lack of direct experimentation and his reliance on pure mathematical reasoning and rational analysis. The more aggressive rejecters of his theory pointed to his Jewish heritage as reason enough to repudiate him.

Of course all that is history, and today Einstein is considered the father of modern physics, and his concepts of relativity are cornerstones of our understanding of our universe; until, of course, another scientist comes along and proves him wrong.

There are many lesser-known mavericks who changed science, people like Ignaz Semmelweis, a 19th-century Hungarian physician. Before the late 1800s a common cause of death among mothers who had recently given birth was puerperal fever, otherwise known as childbed fever. At that time, it was not uncommon for doctors at hospitals to continually shuttle between performing autopsies and attending to women in labour, and not washing their hands between procedures. We may shudder with horror at the thought of it now, but this was a time before the discovery of bacteria. Semmelweis became concerned when his research showed that women who gave birth at home and those who were attended to only by nurses had lower levels of infection than those who gave birth at hospitals where they were attended to by doctors. He concluded that obstetricians who also performed autopsies were transferring what he called 'cadaveric corpuscles' from the bodies of mothers who had died from infection to those who were in labour.

He conducted trials whereby he instructed doctors and medical students in specific labour wards to wash their hands in a chlorine solution before attending to women in labour, and then compared the rates of infection to those where attending staff did not wash their hands. The results, as you can imagine, were clear, but not to his colleagues. The medical fraternity rejected his findings and conclusions, not only because they clashed with conventional medical procedure at that time, but also because they directly implicated doctors in the deaths of their patients. They considered it an affront to their profession. Semmelweis was also unable to provide any scientific *explanation* for his findings.

It wasn't until decades later, when Louis Pasteur developed the concept of germ theory and discovered the pathology of puerperal fever, that Semmelweis was vindicated. By then it was too late for the man who had pioneered the now common medical practice of basic hygiene. Crushed with guilt over his role in the deaths of so many women, rejected and ridiculed by his colleagues, he succumbed to dementia and was admitted to an asylum, where he was bludgeoned to death by guards.

The American biologist and evolutionary theorist Lynn Margulis is another maverick. Back in 1967 she published a paper that proposed that hundreds of millions of years ago, vital structures within eukaryotic cells – those upon which all larger life forms, including you, are based – evolved from simple bacteria when those bacteria formed communities, swapping and merging their genetic codes. To say Margulis's theory of symbiosis in cell evolution was at first met with scorn is an understatement. She was denied funding by the US National Science Foundation for a while, and many fellow biologists rejected her findings with what they considered appropriate scorn. Today her theory is part of mainstream evolutionary biology.

Another maverick who immediately springs to mind – and one closer to Tim Noakes's area of expertise, namely sports science – is Bennet Omalu, the brilliant Nigerian forensic pathologist and neuropathologist who, while working at a Pennsylvania coroner's

I probably saw interviews of him in the PBS documentary "League of denial."

45

These examples of mavericks are good.

2019-04-09
2019-04-09
2019-04-09
2019-04-09
2019-04-09
mitochondria
2019-04-09
2019-04-09
2019-04-09

office in the early 2000s, uncovered a causal link between repeated head injuries in American football players and progressive degeneration of brain function. Omalu's research was central to the identification of what we now call chronic traumatic encephalopathy (CTE). The powerful National Football League (NFL) embarked on a brutal campaign of suppression of Omalu's findings. But eventually, in the face of overwhelming evidence and lawsuits from former players, the NFL was forced to publicly acknowledge the link between concussions sustained in football and CTE. Omalu's story is told in the film *Concussion*, starring Will Smith.

But for pure guts, if you excuse the pun, when it comes to 'good' maverick behaviour in science, the nod has to go to Barry J. Marshall and J. Robin Warren. In the early 1980s, the two Australian researchers were testing an idea that stomach ulcers were caused by bacteria, specifically *Helicobacter pylori*, easily recognisable because of its characteristic flagella – tail-like structures that whip around like rotor blades, helping the bacteria to move. This was a laughable idea at the time, because everyone knew that ulcers were caused by stress and bad eating habits. This meant they could be treated as a chronic – or persistent – condition with any one of a range of gastric interventions sold by pharmaceutical companies. Hundreds of millions of dollars in gastric medication every year depended on this knowledge. It was also believed that the highly acidic environment of the human stomach made it sterile, and therefore a dangerous 'hood for any self-respecting bacteria. And then there was the issue that Marshall and Warren were Australian.

Every time they presented their research, it was met with ridicule. One day, in desperation, after tests with *H. pylori* on pigs failed to produce any result, and after having an endoscopy to ensure he was gastric-ulcer free, Marshall consumed a concoction riddled with the bacteria. If their hypothesis was correct, he believed that, within a few months, he would start developing the characteristic symptoms of a gastric ulcer. He was wrong, but only slightly. Within a matter of days, Marshall felt nauseous, developed halitosis (that would have been courtesy of the bacteria's waste products) and eventually became seriously ill. Follow-up endoscopies and biopsies showed clear evidence of inflammation and damage caused by the bacteria. After treatment with antibiotics, Marshall's health returned. He and Warren then applied their findings by treating patients with gastric ulcers with antibiotics, with similar results. It took a while for their evidence to be accepted by the medical community, but today, for most people, gastric ulcers are not a lifelong curse demanding costly chronic medication; they can be treated with a simple regime of antibiotics. For their research, Marshall and Warren were awarded the Nobel Prize in Physiology or Medicine in 2005. Not bad for a couple of maverick Aussies.

On the other side of the world, it was a couple of Americans who became the poster boys of science obstructionism, earning the sobriquet 'bad' mavericks. They were Frederick Seitz and Fred Singer, both acclaimed Cold War physicists and self-acknowledged free-market fundamentalists, who aligned themselves with various conservative think tanks funded by tobacco, energy and other companies intent on obviating any industrial or environmental federal regulations considered potentially injurious to their business. Among the key areas of scientific consensus that Seitz and Singer focused on disrupting was the link between tobacco smoke and cancer, and, after they lost that battle, anthropogenic climate change. Good use of commas.

What made Seitz and Singer 'obstructionists' was their willingness to step out of academia to embrace corporate interests, and embark on an untethered attack on the integrity of science evolution. Importantly, they didn't challenge science within academia; they took matters out into the public space, relying instead on a programme of targeted media engagement. The purpose was threefold: sow distrust in science, influence public perception and put pressure on regulators.

Seitz, a former president of the US National Academy of Sciences, was recruited by the R.J. Reynolds Tobacco Company in the late 1970s and put in charge of their biomedical research-grant programme. His responsibility was to direct millions of dollars in funding every year to scientists who could be consistently relied on to find no evidence linking tobacco smoke with cancer. He also oversaw an aggressive campaign in the media targeting, often personally, scientists who provided evidence counter to the narrative that R.J. Reynolds and other tobacco companies wanted in the minds of their consumers.

Singer – famously called 'the granddaddy of fake science' by *Rolling Stone* magazine – started his science career in military research with the US Navy, designing mines, before focusing on atmospheric science, where acid rain and the threat of chlorofluorocarbons (CFCs) to the ozone layer were high on his agenda. His libertarian views brought him into conflict with what he perceived were the exorbitantly high costs of addressing the damage to the environment by acid rain and CFCs, and he started becoming an advocate for curbing restrictions on industries contributing to both, considering the environment less important than unencumbered business. He became a darling of libertarian talk shows and right-wing media outlets, such as Fox News and the *National Review*, as well as a key ally of Frederick Seitz.

The negative impacts that the obstructionism of Seitz and Singer have had on the advancement of our understanding of the link between tobacco smoke and cancer, and of the human impact on climate change, are well documented. But if you want to dig deeper into the story, I urge you to read *Merchants of Doubt* by the leading American historians Naomi Oreskes and Erik M. Conway. It is a highly detailed book and the authors researched the matter with due academic diligence and the tenacity of investigative reporters. It uncovers evidence of money-laundering, political arm-wrenching, and programmes of character-assassination aimed at leading scientists who provided the evidence that challenged Seitz and Singer's narrative. Essentially any scientist that strayed from the song sheet was eviscerated.

But damage to the integrity of science by 'bad' mavericks doesn't only come from those engaged in denialism; sometimes it comes from a perfect storm of dodgy science, an errant editorial team and an unquestioning public at the mercy of a media excited by the whiff of hysteria. Case in point: Andrew Wakefield and the MMR vaccine scare.

I am sure that, like me, you have been the beneficiary of the MMR vaccine, normally a combination of two or three jabs given to children before they start attending school, their purpose being to immunise the child against measles, mumps and rubella, three potentially life-threatening diseases. Importantly, the overall efficacy of the MMR vaccine relies on what is known as 'herd or community immunisation' – if sufficient numbers of a community are immunised, it prevents a disease taking any measure of a hold in that community, so it cannot target those who are unable to be immunised, such as children who are too young to be vaccinated, people with immune system problems and those too ill to receive vaccines.

In February 1998, a group of doctors and researchers at the Royal Free Hospital in London published a research paper in *The Lancet,* one of the world's oldest and most respected medical journals. The paper described a study of 12 children who had bowel problems and various perceived behavioural problems,

49

including autism, of which eight of the children had, according to their parents or doctors, developed the symptoms shortly after receiving the MMR vaccine. It's an interesting stretch to link the two, but according to John Snyder, Assistant Professor of Paediatrics at Tufts University School of Medicine and a specialist in medical myths, the researchers claimed that after the children received the MMR vaccine they almost immediately developed a unique bowel disorder, which the researchers later labelled autistic enterocolitis (a term that invites scepticism). They conjectured that as a result of a chronic measles infection induced by the MMR vaccine, which triggered an autoimmune bowel disease that caused their intestines to leak unnamed autism-causing 'toxins', the children had regressed into autism.

The research in the paper was a classic example of what is known as a case series study – as opposed to a cohort study – and it's important to highlight this. Cohort studies are a more robust and analytical form of research and usually follow very strict methodological principles, including the use of control groups, a clearly defined study question, well-described study populations and intervention, validated outcome measures and appropriate statistical analyses, clearly described results and conclusions supported by the data presented, and a complete list of any sources of funding. They are, for the lack of a better word, 'pure' research. Case series studies, however, are more descriptive in their observation and often centre on a single group.

For this reason, and for the fact that the study group was so small, to any pragmatic science journalist such a paper would not be considered newsworthy. That may sound counter-intuitive, but, while the observations were interesting, they were, in effect, anecdotal. The paper itself was, to a degree, circumspect in its language. Given the seriousness of its claim – a possible link between the MMR vaccine and autism – its inclusion in a publication of the calibre of *The Lancet* was puzzling, especially as there was no clear statement of its hypothesis, or conclusions for that matter. It was also clumsily worded in places. That alone should have set alarm bells ringing.

But then things got a little weirder. The hospital called a media conference to announce the findings – which were essentially academic hunches – with the charismatic and media-friendly lead researcher Andrew Wakefield taking centre stage. They suggested that a link had been found between the combination MMR vaccine and autism, and recommended that single vaccines for each of the three diseases were preferable. If such a statement had been made in the halls of academia, there would have been a massive outcry and a stern insistence that the researchers go back to the drawing board and do a far more rigorous cohort study. By going straight to the media with such an explosive summation based on limited research, Wakefield and the hospital were throwing babies to the wolves.

You may be aware of the global fear that subsequently took hold about the safety of the MMR vaccine, and vaccines in general. The fact that Wakefield and his team made a public announcement knowing (a) the limitations of their research and (b) the expected fallout, alone qualifies them for 'bad' maverick status; but, as the marketing saying goes, 'wait, there's more'.

Ironically, the media conference was to be Wakefield's undoing. As the less scientifically literate media ran with the story unchecked, stoking the fires of parental fears, the more inquisitive started asking questions, among them a seasoned investigative reporter for the *Sunday Times* of London, Brian Deer, who had developed a reputation for digging into the medical and pharmaceutical sectors. He reported that Wakefield's study had been sponsored by an attorney hoping to build a case against manufacturers of the MMR vaccine – something that should have been

2019-04-09 disclosed, but wasn't. According to Ben Goldacre in his book *Bad Science*, Wakefield eventually received £435 643 plus expenses from the legal-aid fund set up to develop the case against MMR. Deer also reported that Wakefield had earlier applied for a patent for a test mechanism that relied on showing a link between Crohn's disease – an inflammatory bowel disease – and persisting measles virus infections from vaccines. Any public panic around the MMR vaccine could therefore generate a significant demand for Wakefield's test. Again, this was not disclosed. But what was most distressing was that it seemed many of the children in the study had been subjected to painful and highly invasive procedures, such as colonoscopies and lumbar punches, in order to fulfil the preordained objectives of the study.

Deer's investigation launched demands among regulators for an enquiry into the professional conduct of Wakefield and others associated with the study. In July 2007, over nine years after *The Lancet* published the study paper, the General Medical Council (the British equivalent of the HPCSA that would later investigate Tim Noakes) established a Fitness to Practise Panel that began an enquiry into Wakefield and two other medical professionals associated with the study, Professor John Angus Walker-Smith and Professor Simon Harry Murch. Over a period of two and a 2019-04-09 half years the panel heard from 36 witnesses and deliberated in camera for 45 days before publishing a highly detailed report – the charge sheet runs for 143 pages. It was particularly damning of Wakefield, and pointed out a litany of flaws and biases in his 2019-04-09 research. Brian Deer, later writing in the *British Medical Journal* (*BMJ*), announced the verdict thus: 'It found him guilty of some 30 charges, including four counts of dishonesty and 12 of causing children to be subjected to invasive procedures that were clinically unjustified.' Wakefield and Walker-Smith were eventually struck from the medical registry, Murch was found not guilty, and *The*

Lancet retracted their paper. It was, according to Dr Richard Smith, editor of the *BMJ*, 'the best example there has ever been of a very, very dodgy paper that has created a lot of discomfort and misery'.

Today we thank the stars for those dissident scientists who refused to bend to pressure and remained true to their unconventional insights. Albert Einstein, Ignaz Semmelweis, Lynn Margulis, Bennet Omalu, Barry Marshall and J. Robin Warren were all skilled mavericks who believed passionately about their contradictory theories and in the process shook the science community, but also had the academic capacity and rigour to back up their claims, and were eventually proven correct. Accordingly, they have all been elevated to the status of those who have altered the course of science; they have become game-changers – 'good mavericks'.

But science has also had its fair share of 'bad mavericks': incompetent or fraudulent scientists, and obstructionists, who have floated bizarre theories, or defended corporate interests over public health, usually in the glare of an unquestioning media. Some have been forgotten, but others, like Frederick Seitz, Fred Singer and Andrew Wakefield, have been burnt into the scientific consciousness for the damage they have done.

The question is, if Noakes is indeed a maverick, what type is he?

Chapter 4

A maverick in the ear: Noakes on the sidelines

2019-04-09 Mavericks would not exist if it weren't for herd mentality. As a journalist, I am fascinated with the constructs of social 'conventions' – why most people blindly follow them, but especially why some confidently eschew so-called conventional behaviours. In short, I am intrigued by mavericks.

I have lost count of the number of people who have sat opposite me and replied to a barrage of questions – presidents, politicians, writers, academics, pop stars and other cultural miscreants, sportsmen and women, and other remarkable people – during which time I have become acutely attuned to the subtleties of lying, obfuscation and misrepresentation. I was therefore confident that if I could spend time with Tim Noakes, I could get an idea of what was driving him, and what, if anything, he was hiding.

But I also needed to speak to people who knew him well, but didn't work with him – no one's going to come clean on Professor Noakes if they're going to keep bumping into him in the corridor. They couldn't be family either – Christmas dinners are stressful enough without having to share a turkey drumstick with a turncoat.

I found several willing to speak openly, including one of the world's most famous explorers and extreme athletes, as well as the man *that* Noakes once entrusted to tell his life story. But let's start 2019-04-09 with arguably the most successful coach in the history of Springbok rugby, Jake White.

When White appointed Tim Noakes as official medical consultant to the South African Rugby Union, there was a collective gasp of concern from fans and the media. Here was a man who was no stranger to challenging the sacred conventions of rugby. His first clash was sparked by a tragic event over 20 years earlier, in August 1980: the death of Western Province fullback Chris Burger, following a tackle in a provincial Currie Cup match against Free State. Noakes was listening to the match on the radio and heard the commentator describing Burger being tackled, then collapsing and remaining motionless before being carried off the field, lying face down, on a changing-room door. It emerged that he had received a catastrophic spine injury.

When Burger died the following day, a journalist from the *Sunday Times* contacted Noakes for his reaction. Noakes was a little thrown by being selected for comment, as he had little specific interest in the medical side of rugby – he was a running man – and was certainly no specialist in rugby injuries. But he 2019-04-09 investigated the incident and uncovered several issues that concerned him, including the fact that Burger had not been insured; that there were no facilities at the stadium to deal with such severe injuries; that there was little, if any, specialisation in sports medicine; and that such injuries were quite common in the game, even at school level. This may all sound rather bizarre now, given the intense focus on safety you see in rugby today, but this was 1980 and a different era in rugby. To Noakes at the time it seemed 2019-04-09 that the game's national and provincial governing bodies were mismanaging the safety of their players. So he set about making recommendations for change.

However, it would be a mistake to assume that the game welcomed such changes with any measure of relief, especially via the input of Tim Noakes. At the time of Burger's death, apartheid was still rampant; rugby was played almost entirely by whites and was embraced with an almost religious zeal. Furthermore, the control of rugby was in the hands of a powerful Afrikaans elite who were steadfast in their resistance to change. They were certainly not going to take advice from an English-speaking running doctor with the unfortunate offence of having been born in what was then Rhodesia.

Undeterred, Noakes saw a need to investigate the causes and treatment of spinal injuries, and established a national research programme to study critical rugby injuries, especially those of the spinal cord. The rugby authorities were nonplussed and accused him of interfering, and his calls through the press for more safety in rugby were seen as attempts to 'soften' the game. He did, however, find a powerful ally in former Springbok and Western Province captain Morné du Plessis, who had retired from the game following Burger's death. It was their work together that laid the foundation for the formation – and opening in 1995 in Newlands, Cape Town – of the Sports Science Institute of South Africa. Led by Noakes and Du Plessis, the institute embarked on a campaign to encourage scientific research into rugby injuries.

Today, over 30 years after the death of Chris Burger, professional rugby players are insured; specialised medical teams are on standby at major events; South Africa is a leader in sports science; South African rugby even has its own medical association; and there is ongoing commitment by rugby's international, national and provincial governing bodies to make the game safer, with rules continually being updated to reduce the risk of serious injury.

It was Noakes's contribution to developing the study of the

health and safety of rugby players that made him one of the first to be recruited by Jake White when he was appointed Springbok coach in early 2004. White had inherited a dejected squad, still smarting from being knocked out of the quarter-finals of the 2003 Rugby World Cup and the fallout from the debacle around Kamp Staaldraad (Camp Barbed Wire), a military-styled boot camp during which players were allegedly stripped naked and forced to crawl across gravel, ordered into foxholes, where they were doused with freezing water, and spent nights out in the bush killing chickens. Despite a successful career steering the Springbok Under-21 squad and in various roles with preceding Springbok sides, White was not the first choice for many dedicated South African rugby supporters; their pride was an exposed nerve, and Noakes stepped up to tweak it.

Noakes's recommendation was simple but counter-intuitive: if the Springboks were to win the next Rugby World Cup, in 2007, they had to be prepared to lose. His advice drew from his years working with elite endurance athletes like multi–Comrades Marathon winner Bruce Fordyce. He even invoked the words of Fordyce: 'If you want to be right for the race that really matters, don't try also to be good in the races that are unimportant.' Noakes explained to White the need to rest key players, so that the 22 best players were at peak levels of health and performance going into the World Cup. This meant that there were going to be important games, especially closer to the World Cup, which may have to be sacrificed. For White it was like telling a father to choose which of his children to slaughter.

I managed to track down the former Springbok coach in December 2012 while he was in Zimbabwe on a short break from his commitment to the Brumbies. He smiled when he remembered the ramifications of Noakes's recommendations. 'It may not have been at conflict with me, but I'll tell you what, it was a massive conflict with the people I was working for,' he told me. It was not only the rugby bosses who were riled by the very suggestion of not trying to win every game; fans and the media rose in revolt, too.

Things came to a head in early 2007 during the Tri Nations when, following Noakes's recommendations, White sent a second-string team to play matches in New Zealand and Australia, essentially risking losing all the away fixtures. The media in both countries, and back in South Africa, had a field day, attacking White and his decision; rugby officials in New Zealand and Australia even threatened to scrap their remaining fixtures against the Springboks. The outcome was expected: of the four matches the Springboks played, they lost three and came last in the tournament.

However, three months later they went on to win the Rugby World Cup, and remained the only unbeaten side in the tournament. It's fair to wonder what influence Noakes had on the success outside of his recommendation to rest players. White was emphatic: 'He had a massive influence. I know for a fact that a lot of the medical staff in my team – doctors, physiotherapists, conditioning coaches, anyone with a sports-science link – were in close contact with him all the time.'

But there was another major card that Noakes played that clashed head-on with convention, and one that set the tone for success at the World Cup. Ahead of the tournament, White was under pressure to mentally prepare his team through the rigours of team building. His sights were set on the Olympic Sports Centre in Poland and its famed cryotherapy – brief sessions of exposure to extreme cold. He wanted the whole 'tough love' package: travelling there in economy class, and staying in log cabins as opposed to top hotels. 'I wanted a "come-down-to-earth policy" before building them up.' His alternative was a training camp built around a hike up Mount Kilimanjaro.

White approached Noakes for his recommendation on which one to choose, and Noakes was diplomatically firm in rejecting both: 'Tim said there was no scientific evidence that cryotherapy works to build muscle fitness. It may work psychologically, but that is the equivalent of a placebo. He dismissed it as a lot of money to take them away to boost them psychologically.' Regarding an expedition to climb Kilimanjaro, Noakes warned White that after spending months building up their bodies and strength, such a trip could see them lose an average of five kilograms each. 'And don't forget,' he told White, 'someone could die.'

Noakes's alternative recommendation flew in the face of the established tradition of hard knocks, embraced so disastrously at Kamp Staaldraad: 'Keep them at home, let them relax and spend time with their families.' As an extension to the policy of resting key players, it made sense. 'But let me say this,' White insisted, 'if he had said cryotherapy is the way to go, and that not only will it have psychological benefits, but it's scientifically proven to improve the players' physical strength and performance, then I would have gone hammer and tongs across to Poland.'

White emphasised that Noakes's recommendations were instrumental in the Springboks' clear record in the 2007 Rugby World Cup: 'I have no doubt that by not going to Poland, we had an opportunity to get other things right. The fact that those boys didn't go to the Tri Nations, and therefore didn't have to travel ahead of the World Cup, was for them a boost because they could spend time with their families.' This meant for the two weeks before the start of the World Cup, they could concentrate on preparing themselves ahead of two of their hardest games: England and Samoa.

In retrospect it's easy to say that Noakes was right; but it's also easy to forget that at that time almost every major recommendation he made to White was castigated by a dogmatic rugby union, and scrutinised and often criticised by an all-knowing media

2019-04-09

Related to the title of this chapter.

2019-04-09

feeding the voracious appetite of a rugby-loving nation entrenched in a win-at-all-costs mentality. Noakes was often portrayed as a Lady Macbeth figure, capitalising on enjoying the ear of the Springbok coach by whispering all manner of pernicious encouragement, all the time bent on personal aggrandisement.

2019-04-09

Reminding White of this, I was intrigued with how he justified embracing the scientific opinion of one person against that of his superiors and, seemingly, the entire nation. 'I had full faith in what Tim said, because I knew he genuinely wanted South Africa to win. I always had the feeling in every meeting that we had that he genuinely wanted to find ways in which we could have the edge over the opposition. And he never gave me a reason to doubt him.'

2019-04-09

So was Noakes challenging the status quo because he was excited to push the frontiers of science in sport, or did he seem to get a kick out of shaking things up? White insisted that Noakes was always composed when providing input, and that he had a quiet authority about him: 'He never said to us, don't do it like that, do it like this. He always gave you options and the pros and cons of both options.'

2019-04-09

This would have resonated with his role as a sports scientist, and suggests that his recommendations were always measured and the impacts calculated. More importantly, insisted White, he had a quality that's rare in sport management: he was comfortable with challenging his own counsel. 'It's that intrinsic belief that if you want to find the leading edge in sports science, you have to test theories and challenge principles, even your own,' said White. 'And he's brave enough to do it.'

Finally, added White, it was while working with the Springboks that Noakes discovered a part of himself that he didn't know existed: 'He has a wonderful gut feel about being a coach. When you're a coach, you have to adapt on your feet. If coaching was as easy as having a recipe which you then give to someone and they go off and do it, then everyone would be doing it.'

The themes of making careful calculated decisions, challenging what others deemed convention and combining them to coach others to push things to the very edge would prove to be successful in another of Noakes's ventures; one that may not have been with rugby, but which nevertheless involved some pretty big balls. It was also one that could have gone disastrously wrong.

slang. [2019-0409]

There's a joke that no self-respecting man swims in the sea off Cape Town wearing a Speedo, for fear of evident shrinkage. The cold Benguela Current that forms off the Cape of Good Hope and moves northwards up the west coast of southern Africa draws from the South Atlantic cold, nutrient-rich water that brushes up against Antarctica. The result is that the warm golden sands of Cape Town's beaches dip invitingly into a sea that is best explored wearing a full wetsuit.

But that's not the only reason *that* the seas off Cape Town challenge those who enter it. Where the Benguela starts, it rubs shoulders with the powerful Agulhas Current, which drags warm, volatile equatorial water down the east coast. The result is a mercurial and complex weather pattern above it that has blessed the coast with a rich floral heritage, but made charting the coastline a nightmare. Violent storms and powerful currents test even the most seasoned mariner, and those who fail become another of the many shipwrecks that scatter the coastline of the Cape of Good Hope.

20190409

And yet it was in these seas that Lewis Gordon Pugh sought to take part in a solo marathon swim, wearing nothing but a Speedo.

2019-0409

Pugh is not normal; in fact, he is nothing short of extraordinary. His capacity to raise his core body temperature at will – a conditioned response called anticipatory thermogenesis – means that he is capable of swimming in extremely cold water. He is every bit an extreme athlete, continually pushing the boundaries

2019-0409

of what his mind and body are capable of, and in the process, has become an active environmental activist, using high-profile swimming expeditions to highlight his campaigns.

It seems no swim is beyond his mettle. He found the English Channel akin to a walk in the park, and was the first to complete long-distance swims in every ocean. When, in 2004, he decided he wanted to swim around the Cape Peninsula, a distance of 100 kilometres, he found no friend or fellow swimmer who thought it possible. Not only had the gale-force winds and building-high waves claimed the lives of hundreds of sailors, but the bitterly cold waters were also home to sharks and other predators that would willingly pick off anyone foolish enough to dip their toe in.

With naysayers claiming there was no way he could do it, he went to the one person who had experience working with athletes under extreme conditions, albeit runners exposed to heat, and asked him if his body could handle it. 'Yes,' said Noakes, without hesitation. He then went on to explain that if Pugh had the mind to do it, his body would follow, something on which Noakes had become a world authority; and recommended a focused training regime that would help prepare him.

After successfully completing the Cape Peninsula swim, Pugh considered pushing the limits even further, and approached Noakes for help with what was going to be the first of a number of swims in increasingly cold water. It was the start of a highly successful relationship between scientist and subject, and eventually coach and athlete, that could have ended in tragedy, but instead culminated in a swim that defied logic and convention.

The first project with Noakes as scientist and part of the support team was a one-kilometre swim in the sea off Spitsbergen, an island midway between Norway and the North Pole and which borders the Arctic Ocean, where the sea temperature is less than four degrees Celsius. As a matter of comparison, the sea off Cape

Town rarely drops below 12 degrees at its coldest. The second consisted of two swims off the Antarctic Peninsula, where the water drops to zero degrees – a one-kilometre swim off Petermann Island and a 1.6-kilometre swim in the waters of Port Foster, a bay within the horseshoe-shaped Deception Island – and the third a swim in an open stretch of sea at the geographic North Pole in water that was minus 1.7 degrees Celsius.

So why would Noakes, a physiologist specialising in runners, want to help a swimmer subject himself to freezing cold water? Was he attracted to the thrill of it, the ghoulish spectre of physical risk, or did he want to poke convention in the eye and watch it shudder? I put the question to Pugh while he was taking a well-deserved break from environmental campaigning. He laughed off any suggestion of an over-adventuresome motive; instead, he explained that Noakes had done a lot of studies of athletes operating under conditions of extreme heat – dehydration and over-hydration – and this was an opportunity to examine an athlete working at the other extreme. 'Now he could see the opposite side of the spectrum, and get a full understanding of thermoregulation: from extreme cold to extreme heat. It was invaluable.'

I suggested that it must have been great for a scientist like Noakes to tag along for the ride. Pugh was quick to clarify that that was not the case: 'He was mission critical.' Pugh explained that Noakes was not only intimately involved in his preparation and training for every endeavour, but he was also continually monitoring and supporting him during the swim, usually right next to him in a boat. Pugh pointed out that his health and well-being was always of primary concern to Noakes: 'Everything was about safety, safety, safety. I would never have had the confidence to get in the water had he not been there. None of these swims would have been possible without him.'

Pugh admitted that there was a brief moment at first when he felt like a subject in a scientific experiment, and still smiles when he reads himself described as such in the scientific papers Noakes published from their collaboration; but he soon realised that even though Noakes approached the swims with the discipline of a scientist, he embraced Pugh's passion for shattering convention. This became evident when one of the swims nearly ended in tragedy.

Halfway through the swim off Petermann Island, with Pugh's support team in a boat next to him, they were hit by an unexpected snowstorm. Noakes's responsibility was to carefully monitor Pugh's vital signs, such as heart rate and core body temperature, via a series of sensors in and on his body and a transmitter strapped to his back, and immediately pull Pugh out should they drop to dangerous levels. Under such extreme conditions, hesitation, mistiming or miscalculation could be fatal. The information was also fed to an assistant, who would write it on a whiteboard and show it to Pugh as his head turned out of the water. Pugh remembered glancing up to see Noakes hunched over his laptop: 'Snow was piling up on his eyebrows. He looked like Father Christmas.'

However, the driving snow also made the whiteboard slippery, and the assistant dropped the pen and watched helplessly as it got lost in the boat. During the confusion, Pugh looked up to see no updates on the board and started panicking. Sensing Pugh's desperation and knowing how critically he needed the information, Noakes stood up and started shouting, above the roar of the wind and the noise of the boat's motor, how Pugh was doing and how far he had left, encouraging him with every stroke. Pugh said it was an event that sparked a shift in their collaboration: 'That was a crucial moment when Tim changed from being a scientist to being a coach.'

That was the second reference to 'coach', and I asked Pugh if it meant a change in Noakes's approach, a slackening of the equable 'scientist' and an embracing of a more excitable attitude to the task at hand. Pugh shook his head: 'He's never, ever been reckless. He never fired from the hip. Everything from him was a considered view.' He said that even though Noakes embraced the challenge of the boundaries set by convention, he always understood the risk, and approached each task with the discipline of a scientist. 'He would always ask us what assumptions we were making and are they valid,' Pugh told me. I drew a big circle around that point in my notes, sensing it was a key component to the story that was unfolding, a possible philosophical attribute of a maverick.

Pugh emphasised that the risk was not only his every time, and this was especially the case during the Arctic swim. He remembered a moment just before they were to get off the ship and into the water for the swim. The water was completely black, almost like an inkpot. 'Tim was strapping the measuring equipment onto my body, and as he was doing it, I could feel his hands shaking. When one of the world's top doctor's hands are shaking, you begin to wonder if you're doing the right thing. And it was only at that moment that I realised what I was putting him through as well. I looked him straight in the eye and said to him, "Tim, I just want you to know how very grateful I am to you, because there are not many doctors who would be prepared to assume this much risk." And he looked at me and said quietly, confidently and without hesitation, "Lewis, I wouldn't miss this. Now let's go and do it."'

Pugh paused for a minute as if reminded of what had been at stake. 'Imagine if I hadn't have come back. Everyone would be looking at Tim differently now, very differently. He was the guy who took the swimmer to the North Pole, and the swimmer died. I may be the one who would lose my life, but he's the one who would have to look everyone in the eye.'

As our interview drew to a close, Pugh reminded me of all the other doctors and specialists whom he had asked who refused to help, pointing out that they had all said that they were simply not comfortable with the responsibility of taking on such a challenge and the reputational ramifications if things were to go wrong. 'The world,' said Pugh, 'is divided into pioneers and followers. Tim will never be a follower.'

'Would you say he's a maverick?' I asked Lewis. Again, the pause. His answer intrigued me. It seemed in part contradictory, but at the same time, in a way, quite apt. I scribbled it down, then circled it, thinking it may deserve re-examining later.

Just as helping a swimmer in the extreme cold or setting a training agenda for a team of rugby players may seem at odds for a physiologist and researcher specialising in the performance of runners in extreme heat, so must writing about that physiologist be for a sports journalist more at ease writing about golf. But Michael Vlismas, the co-author with Noakes of *Challenging Beliefs: Memoirs of a Career*, is no stranger to rubbing shoulders with sporting mavericks. In 2010 he published *Don't Choke: A Champion's Guide to Winning Under Pressure* with Gary Player. A veteran sports journalist and broadcaster, and editor of a golfing magazine, Vlismas seemed the ideal choice to team up with one of the world's greatest golfers and a thorn in the side of convention. Now in his eighties, Player refuses to retire like other men his age, and instead still plays competitive golf, follows a demanding training regime, and runs a global business empire, as well as various academies and charity organisations.

I thought that if anyone could give me a closer look at Tim Noakes and what drives him to challenge convention, it would be his biographer. So I tracked him down and asked him if there were any similarities of character between Noakes and Gary Player. Vlismas seemed intrigued by the question, as if he'd never really

66

considered it, before answering: 'Both of them believe in the power of the mind. Gary has an unshakeable belief that if he puts his mind to something, he will achieve it – and he does. In that respect, he's an absolute machine. Tim understands this and can obviously explain the science behind it.'

Having said that, I suspected that they were different characters. Vlismas agreed: 'Tim has a quiet energy about him, while Gary is right out there – he's in your face. People have called him self-promoting, but as he's always said, no one's going to get more excited about you than yourself, so you might as well do so. Tim is very humble, very down to earth, and has a quieter drive than Gary Player; but they both share a horror at injustice in the world. Tim is shocked with the levels of corruption in sport. It genuinely affects him. A lot of us may say that's life and just carry on, but Tim insists that it's not right. It's as if his value system is a lot more evolved than that of most people.'

It made sense that if this was the case, then what Noakes said and did would rub some people up the wrong way, perhaps clash with conventional opinion. Vlismas agreed with my summation: 'Absolutely. People find him an antagonist – "Oh, there's Tim Noakes meddling again."' He then proceeded to provide examples of when Noakes had stuck his nose in where others felt it didn't belong: 'For example, when he took on rugby [after the death of Chris Burger], it was a fine line. When he was saying, you have to change the laws of the tackle and at the breakdown to make it safer for school kids, [then South African Rugby Board president] Danie Craven and the rugby authorities saw him as meddling in the sport; whereas all he was saying was, "I'm not meddling in rugby, I love rugby. I just want to make it safer."'

Vlismas also reminded me that Noakes was one of the first to publicly voice the opinion that cricket in South Africa was riddled with corruption. 'He did so because he loved cricket. He just wanted to highlight that it was damaging the game.' He was later proven correct.

But, as Vlismas explained, even the most virtuous of intentions didn't cushion Noakes when his research and findings undermined the supposedly secure foundations of the billion-dollar bottom line of a powerful multinational corporate brand: Gatorade.

In the early 1980s, Noakes's research into the performance of runners in extreme heat had uncovered a distressing paradox: athletes were showing the symptoms of heatstroke and dehydration, even though they were consuming plenty of water. He suspected that these athletes were in fact consuming *too much* water and were developing hyponatremia, or over-hydration, where the sodium levels in the blood drop to below normal levels, resulting in nausea, vomiting, headaches, muscle spasms and fatigue – similar symptoms to the polar opposite condition of dehydration.

The term 'exercise-associated hyponatremia', or EAH, was coined and Noakes went about investigating it further, resulting in his publication in 1985 of a paper in the journal *Medicine & Science in Sports & Exercise* titled 'Water intoxication: A possible complication during endurance exercise'. It described the occurrence of hyponatremia in four athletes who had participated in endurance events that were longer than seven hours. It would be the first of many papers he'd publish that would drive research in what would become a developing area of sports medicine.

But there was a problem. What Noakes was suggesting clashed with the so-called science of hydration that had been championed by the US-based food conglomerate Quaker Oats Company, who owned the popular sports drink Gatorade. There's an entertaining aside here that warrants telling. The original formula behind

68

Gatorade was developed by three University of Florida–based doctors, J. Robert Cade, Dana Shires and Alejandro de Quesada. Cade was a kidney specialist and intent on designing a fluid to provide a healthy balance of water, carbohydrates and electrolytes to replace those lost by the university students during sport. When the formula was completed, according to records, one of the members of his team claimed it tasted like toilet-bowl cleaner, and when Cade tried it, he immediately threw up. The formula was bought by an Indianapolis-based canned food company called Stokely-Van Camp, who had to dramatically dilute and reformulate it before branding it as Gatorade.

In 1985, the Quaker Oats Company, having bought Stokely-Van Camp two years earlier, were in the throes of a major marketing offensive and saw Gatorade as a shining light in their stable. They wanted to herald the virtues of Gatorade, that it replaced valuable salts and minerals lost through perspiration when exercising.

They sought to underpin this assertion by using science, and so embarked on a drive to associate Gatorade with sports science by throwing money behind associations such as the Australian Institute of Sport and the American College of Sports Medicine (ACSM). Shortly after receiving funding, the ACSM published drinking guidelines in sport that were extremely advantageous to Gatorade, with associate spikes in sales. The overall effect was also a burgeoning belief within sport that continual hydration, especially with sports drinks, would prevent dehydration and the reduction of sodium levels in the blood.

However, nutrition, biology and basic chemistry held evidence to counter the claims of the industry-sponsored 'science of hydration': firstly, a typical Western diet contains high levels of salt, meaning that most athletes on such a diet would retain more than enough sodium in their blood to cover any losses through exercise. Secondly, humans have retained highly effective salt-conserving mechanisms as a throwback from our earlier days wandering the African savannah. Thirdly, the concentration of sodium in most sports drinks, including Gatorade, is microscopic, about 20 mmol/L (millimoles per litre), whereas in blood a healthy concentration is around 140 mmol/L. In effect, this means that any time you drink a sports drink, you are essentially diluting your blood sodium concentration, unless your body has regulatory mechanisms to prevent this.

When it came to studying exercise-associated hyponatremia, Noakes clashed with other researchers in sports science for two reasons: firstly, a lot of research into EAH, especially in the US, was being conducted in laboratories where variables could be controlled to help ensure a predetermined outcome, and where athletes were generally tested for a maximum of eight hours at a time. Noakes's research, however, was mainly conducted in the field, during competition, where triathletes can compete for anywhere up to 17 hours. Secondly, scientists who were enjoying financial support from Gatorade dominated the editorial boards of most of the leading publications in the exercise sciences, and what Noakes's research was suggesting flew in the face of what Gatorade was hoping to establish as scientific consensus.

As a result, Noakes was vilified in, what he claims, was a highly elaborate, industry-sponsored campaign designed to question his research and damage his reputation. Extensive work done in South Africa on fluid and exercise and understanding EAH remained out of major exercise science journals, and Noakes was shunned from beverage industry–sponsored sports and exercise conventions. During this time there was a noticeable increase in incidences of EAH in various running and sporting events, resulting in a number of deaths. It wasn't until 2007 that the ACSM acknowledged that the research on EAH driven by Noakes was correct, and responded by introducing new guidelines support-

ing the research that athletes should only drink according to the 2019-04-09
dictates of thirst.

Even though Noakes and the developing corps of sports scientists who showed the dangers of over-drinking emerged, at least
in part, victors in the scrap with the Quaker Oats Company and
later PepsiCo, which bought out Quaker Oats, it left Noakes with 2019-04-09
a sobering lesson: If you challenge convention when big money 2019-04-09
is at stake, things will get nasty.

So why did he carry on? I put this question to Vlismas, who
smiled and said that he had asked Noakes the same thing. 'I just
didn't like the way the manufacturers of Gatorade were "milking" 2019-04-09
the game for financial gain and confusing people and contributing to their ill-health as a result of over-hydrating,' Noakes
told him, before adding, 'Besides, I love endurance sport and
examining how the body operates under stress.'

But there was an element to the story of Noakes's fight with 2019-04-09
Gatorade that left me feeling a little uneasy, even doubtful. In
Challenging Beliefs, reference is made to the 'Mafia of Science',
and claims are made that Gatorade infiltrated the very bastion
of scientific theory – the peer-review system. The book suggests
that the system was manipulated by the sports-drink manufac-
turer to, in effect, censure any research, including Noakes's, that
questioned the prevailing science of hydration.

I put to Vlismas that it left me with the impression that Noakes
was toying with conspiracy theories, hardly the realm of the serious scientist. He agreed that such an impression was logical, but
then explained how it was part of Noakes's research repertory:
'As a journalist you're trained to look right through conspiracy 2019-04-09
theories, and so there were often times when I thought, "Come
on, you can't be serious", and Tim admitted that initially when
such an idea came into his head it seemed a little unbelievable, 2019-04-09
but that he would then think, let's investigate this and see where

it goes. And as absurd and off the charts as it may have seemed, he would invariably be proven correct.'

I pushed Vlismas on the matter of a 'Mafia of Science', and he replied in a prescient tone, 'It may be a few years, even a decade or two, but he'll be proven right.'

So was Noakes right in the latest fight, that with nutritionists? Should we re-examine the current prevailing models of nutrition? Vlismas pointed to the continual quest of science for veracity and adjustment, and how Noakes seemed to be its embodiment: 'He is driven by the integrity of the scientific process, and that if you get a result, to examine why you get that result. If we get a model that says that A+B=C, then we need to make sure that in 10 years' time A+B still equals C, and that if it doesn't, then we need to relook that model.'

Even if it means challenging the scientific status quo? Did Noakes genuinely believe that science would always reject faulty data or manipulated results? Vlismas laughed, and suggested Noakes's passion for the self-correcting integrity of science ran deep: 'You know, I think he honestly gets turned on by it.'

I thought it a rather provocative statement about someone supposedly immersed in the serious endeavour of scientific know-ledge, but it suggested that there was indeed something that may set him apart from other scientists I had interviewed. There was only one way to find out. It was time to meet Professor Tim Noakes.

72

Chapter 5

Noakes on Noakes

Nestled below Cape Town's Table Mountain and, quite aptly, between the famous twin monuments to Western Province sport – Newlands rugby and cricket stadia – is the Sports Science Institute of South Africa. Originally designed as a facility to fund research and apply it to sport, today it houses a high-performance centre, a wellness centre and numerous specialised health service clinics, all offering programmes to professional and non-professional athletes. It also provides scores of education, training and social-investment outreach programmes.

Arguably, though, its most valuable asset is on the third floor: the University of Cape Town Research Unit for Exercise Science and Sports Medicine. It is the home of some of the world's most cutting-edge research into sports medicine. At the time of my first interview for this book, on 11 December 2012, Professor Tim Noakes was head of the unit, and it is here where he was based.

To say Noakes is a highly qualified, globally respected academic and teacher, and no intellectual slouch, is unquestionably an understatement; and this is spelled out by the trail of letters after his name: OMS, MBChB, MD, DSc, PhD (hc), FACSM, (hon) FFSEM (UK), (hon) FFSEM (Ire). This means he has been awarded a Bachelor of Medicine, Bachelor of Surgery, Doctor of Medicine,

Doctor of Science and Honorary Doctor of Philosophy; and that he is a Fellow of the American College of Sports Medicine and an Honorary Fellow of the Faculty of Sport and Exercise Medicine in both the UK and Ireland. The OMS is something of which he is especially proud – it's the Order of Mapungubwe, Silver, South Africa's highest civil honour, awarded to Noakes for his contribution to exercise science and sports medicine.

He has also been accorded the highest National Research Foundation (NRF) rating for a scientist – A1 – meaning that, according to the NRF, he is recognised as a leading scholar in his field internationally for the high quality and wide impact of his recent research outputs. This is evident in the fact that he has been cited more than 12 500 times in scientific literature.

But it's in Noakes's CV that the real wealth of his impact on exercise science and sports medicine can be fully appreciated. Sticking to only the fundamentals of academic requirements, such as the titles and references of published peer-reviewed articles and letters (almost 500 in total), other published articles, titles of talks presented at international conventions, and lists of postgraduate PhD theses that he has supervised, it still stretches to 77 pages. For the more pedantic reader, that's in single-spaced Arial font size 11.

This made it a little strange when I finally met Noakes. Expecting to find a soberly dressed, pensive academic with formidable gravitas, I was pleasantly surprised to discover instead a sprightly, beaming, slightly boyish man, fully at home popping in and out of offices wearing shirt, slacks and running shoes. But then, as someone explained later, 'that's Tim'.

His office spoke volumes about his studiousness – the shelves behind and around his desk groaned under the weight of books and research papers, and yet there still seemed plenty of space for various sporting awards and sentimental bric-a-brac.

The day of our interview was typical of a Cape Town summer: hot and dry with little chance of rain; and yet Noakes preferred to renounce the comfort of air-conditioning to sit with the window open, as if not wanting to shut himself off from the sporting heritage within touching distance outside. The warm wind that rolled inside carried with it the heavy, heady aroma from the nearby brewery. I thought it cruelly ironic that the office of a man who had dedicated his life to the health of sportsmen and women should be drenched in the aromatic residue of a product that has such a damaging influence on the health and lives of so many people.

'We meet at last,' I said, alluding to the flow of emails between our offices and the hasty rescheduling of a previous meeting. We had been set to meet five days earlier, the day of the debate with Jacques Rossouw, and I now suggested that given his state of mind ahead of it, it was no wonder he had wanted to reschedule. He nodded, smiled and explained that for weeks before the debate he had thought of nothing else, becoming quite stressed in the process, and that he was glad it was finally over.

The smile seemed to hide the hurt I'd seen develop during the debate, especially in the question session that followed so abruptly after Rossouw's presentation. There was supposed to have been a rebuttal from Noakes, but it never happened. I asked Noakes why. He sighed and shook his head rather angrily, 'I withdrew from that because I realised it was a witch-hunt, a kangaroo court. It wasn't a debate. I realised the audience wasn't constructive; that anything I said was seen as inflammatory. So I just decided that's it.'

I gathered I had struck a nerve and decided to shift the tone, but made a note to return to investigate it.

It made sense to start at the beginning, and suspecting that a clue to his penchant for bucking trends lay in his upbringing,

I asked if that were the case. His eyes looked upwards and a goofy smile burst across his face. 'I am sure there's some type of obscure reason connected with the fact that I was sent to boarding school at the age of seven,' he said. 'That had a deep effect on me, because I was wrenched from my mother at such a young age. I was incredibly close to my mother, and I never really repaired that relationship. I couldn't understand what I had done wrong to be thrown out of the house. It was probably the right thing, but it had consequences.' He admitted that the feelings of rejection had probably manifested themselves in an undercurrent of defiance against what he saw as 'authority': 'I think I've always been raging against that – it's a rage – a quiet rage I haven't resolved; and I don't pretend to understand it, but at least I'm dealing with it in a positive manner.'

If that were the case, then science, given its proclivity towards establishing authority, was not a prudent choice for a person with his character inclination. Surely he was setting himself up for confrontation? He nodded, almost retrospectively. 'I can't stand people who have no creativity, no imagination, who can't think that there must be another way,' he admitted. 'I find that so frustrating. And unfortunately that's the case with so many people in my discipline. Ninety per cent of the scientists I know don't like change – they want to go to work, do their job and go home at night. They don't want to change the world.'

Therein, it seemed, lay part of the formula for the sequence of events that had found Noakes on the receiving end of so much rebuke, and, in a way, may have explained his choice of sports science. When Noakes was a student, sports medicine was something of a Cinderella science – all pretty and sparkly, but it certainly wasn't a direction to be taken seriously. Noakes explained that when he was studying medicine, he saw three major problems, all of which related back to the topic of our discussion:

'Firstly, there was no interest in health – it was all about disease treatment; secondly, it was completely cost-ineffective; and, thirdly, they didn't care a damn about athletes.' Like most of his research, there was a personal point of entry: 'So when I got injured, there was no one who could help me.'

There was another reason that he turned his back on the traditional direction of medicine – patient care and surgery – which shows an element of his personality that he normally keeps hidden: 'Medicine is emotionally very demanding, and I didn't have the emotional strength to deal with the potential death of patients.'

I sensed that there was something more to his choice of sports medicine besides the avoidance of the expected heartache of losing patients. Surely it was something about sport, perhaps a parallel with science? The smile returned. 'Absolutely. The beauty of sport is that you have to address questions every week, and if you don't address them, you just become irrelevant.'

He paused as if he were then putting on his scientist's cap. 'In science, it's the same: there's always a measurement – your next scientific paper. That's a measure of where you've gone over the last few months, and you can see a process of building on those papers. The thing about science is that at the end of the day, you know just how good a scientist is – just as you can tell how good an athlete is – by their performance in relation to the rest of the world.'

There is, of course, a difference: whereas the travails and performance of sportsmen and women is public and easily accessible – splashed all over the media – the delivery and accomplishment of scientists – their research – is often locked away in journals, away from easy public access and camouflaged by layers of data and technical jargon.

It seems, now, quite prophetic that Noakes's first such research was also the first to see him clash with hallowed medical beliefs.

77

It was 1976, and Noakes had just started his research career at UCT under Professor Lionel Opie. He came across research by a California-based physician, Dr Tom Bassler, that suggested that marathon runners didn't die of coronary atherosclerosis, a disease of the heart characterised by a hardening of the artery walls as they become thickened with a waxy substance called plaque, resulting in a reduction of the flow of oxygen-rich blood to the heart.

Bassler's findings were based on an autopsy done on 70-year-old Clarence DeMar, a legendary American marathon runner who had died of cancer, which showed that the diameter of his coronary arteries was two to three times the normal size. In addition, he had almost no atherosclerotic plaque. Bassler also battled to find a single documented case of a marathon runner who had died of coronary atherosclerosis. He considered this evidence sufficient to support his theory that marathon runners were somehow immune to coronary artery disease. It was a rather enthusiastic leap of logic. It was also highly contagious, and helped kick-start a surge in interest in running, especially in the US.

Noakes found the suppositions of Bassler's research intriguing, and his suspicion that they were faulty spurred him to trawl the country looking at autopsies of runners who had died of a suspected heart attack. His research also uncovered two veteran marathon runners who had survived heart attacks. Tests on them showed unequivocal evidence of coronary atherosclerosis.

Armed with his findings, Noakes flew to the US to hastily address a special conference on marathon running being held by the New York Academy of Sciences. The conference had been arranged to celebrate the New York City Marathon, ironically one of the outcomes of this new popular running craze. Noakes had a dual agenda: he was also there to run the marathon.

As luck, or misfortune, would have it, Dr Bassler was also scheduled to address the conference; and so, at the relatively young age of 27, Noakes stood up before the pantheon of American exercise physiology and sports medicine and provided evidence to refute the findings of one of its most exalted members, who also just happened to be in the audience. At the same time, he sounded a wake-up call for the thousands of runners who were about to run 42 kilometres, believing, incorrectly, that in doing so they were immune to developing a disease of the arteries. It was Noakes's first step towards shaking some fundamental beliefs of modern science.

He nodded reminiscently when I reminded him of his first brush with medical authority, and the hackles that were raised at his perceived imprudence. 'It's not as if I went out to rock convention,' he said. 'Tom Bassler's theory was based on an absence of evidence; that is, since there was no record of a marathon runner dying from coronary atherosclerosis, all runners must be immune. I knew it was only a matter of time before a careful hunt would find the first marathon runner to die from that disease.' Importantly, he was right.

That was four decades ago, and he's still chipping away at the canons of accepted medicine around coronary heart disease. However, he's no longer a brash upstart; he's a far better scientist, a lot better read, and a lot wiser. He has also secured a remarkable track record of being proven correct, and in changing mindsets about fundamentals of exercise science and sports medicine. You could argue that this should have given his latest challenge more immediate credence, and suggest it be embraced with at least an open mind.

However, things were a little different this time. He had stepped out of the field of exercise science and further into nutrition. One of his detractors, a leading academic in dietetics who wished to remain anonymous, had told me that Noakes had taken a step too far. She dismissed as 'irresponsible' his charge that conventional nutritional guidelines recommending a low-fat, high-carbohydrate diet posed a serious risk to people predisposed to diabetes, saying that because he had been researching the topic for only two years, he was not qualified to talk on nutrition and should 'go back to sports medicine'.

Noakes chuckled when I brought this up. Sweeping an arm around his office, he explained that in those two years he had not only read almost 70 books on the varying benefits of low-fat, high-carbohydrate diets and low-carbohydrate, high-fat, high-protein diets, but had also critically analysed reams of research on insulin resistance and type 2 diabetes, and their association with heart disease and other chronic health problems. 'What I've learnt over the last two years,' he said, 'is that 80 per cent of chronic ill-health is nutrition-based.' He threw up his arms in mock surprise, 'But this is not taught. Why is it not taught? Because people don't understand it.'

'Are you misunderstood?' I asked Noakes. He shook his head. 'They say I'm wrong because they say saturated fats cause levels of cholesterol to increase and that cholesterol causes heart disease.' The solution then proffered by medicine, he explained, was the prescription of statins – a class of medicine designed to lower blood cholesterol levels, and a multibillion-dollar industry.

'But the problem is when you take the fat out of the diet and put the carbohydrate in, you get a whole bunch of other diseases. And they don't recognise that. They think there's only one disease you die from, and that's heart disease. But people also die of cancer of the colon and cancer of the breast, both of which are carbohydrate-dependent diseases. They get dementia, which is a carbohydrate-dependent disease; they get a whole bunch of diet disorders, which are cereal- and grain-based disorders; and there are also allergic and immune diseases which are related to [the consumption of] cereals and grains.'

'Perhaps they are right and you are wrong?' I suggested. 'You've been wrong before.' He knew I was referring to his former encouragement of carbo-loading ahead of marathons. He shook his head. 'When I wrote *Lore of Running*, what I wrote on carbs was received wisdom – I received it from other people – and I was reporting on what was said by scientists.' He was referring to some of those whom he was now challenging, this time armed with detailed research of his own.

2019-04-09

He then returned to what he saw was another fundamental flaw in health care and the teaching of medicine: that the focus is on the disease, not the patient. He quoted one of the founding professors of Johns Hopkins Hospital, Sir William Osler, who was renowned for his pithy take on the teaching of medicine: 'The good physician treats the disease; the great physician treats the patient who has the disease.'

2019-04-09

'Their model,' said Noakes, referring to the current medical teaching establishment, 'is that for each disease there's a different drug.' I paused as what he was saying began to sink in. I raised a finger. 'But then what you're saying is threatening entire industries – those associated with treating diseases that could be prevented through proper nutrition.' He nodded, shrugged and smiled somewhat sadly, 'Exactly.'

2019-04-09
2019-04-09

This was bigger than challenging a foundation of nutrition. This was about upending the fundamentals of medical training. He could see the realisation on my face, smiled and slowly shook his head. 'We're not teaching prevention,' he said. I asked him why this was. 'Because the pharmaceutical industry runs what is taught in the medical schools because they control the specialists, and they entice the specialists to believe that the drugs are the only way to go.' I shifted uneasily in my chair, uncomfortable with another allusion to conspiracy within the ranks of medicine.

2019-04-09

But then I remembered something that Glen Hagemann had told

2019-04-09

81

me. Hagemann is the former president of the South African Sports Medicine Association, a multidisciplinary association for any medical professionals who have an interest in sports medicine, including biokineticists, sport physicians, physiotherapists and dietitians. When I asked him why there seemed to be such an outpouring of outrage from the medical community, and specifically dietitians and nutritionists, towards Noakes's claims, he said, 'There's no doubt it's a threat to their livelihood. It challenges the very fundamentals of what they've been taught and what they are teaching. It's almost like a doctor being told that Western medicine is absolute rubbish. It's demanding a complete paradigm shift.'

Then I remembered something else Hagemann had said that made me want to revisit that nerve I had tweaked in the beginning of the interview with Noakes, and which could possibly explain the hostility at the debate. Hagemann explained that it was known that when Noakes tackled an issue, he was clearly onto something, that he had done his research, and that, like a terrier, he wasn't going to let go. 'Being one of the top research scientists in his field, he is able to recognise "bad science" and tear studies apart that are not methodologically sound,' Hagemann explained. 'Unfortunately, too many decisions are commercially based and founded on "bad science", and he is not afraid to confront this issue.'

In the debate, Noakes claimed that a landmark study that was part of the Women's Health Initiative, which his challenger, Dr Jacques Rossouw, had overseen, actually supported his central argument that a high-carbohydrate diet produced dangerous, high-level spikes of insulin in those people with a predisposition towards diabetes, and contributed to the development of coronary heart disease. However, according to Noakes, even though this was a critical discovery, because it clashed with the fundamentals of so-called traditional nutritional guidelines, it was not highlighted. In fact, Noakes claimed, not only was the evidence left buried within the data, but that data was then also misrepresented. Was this the type of 'bad science' Hagemann had been talking about?

Noakes's anger flared again when I brought it up. 'All [Rossouw] could say was that it was a printer's error. Bullshit it's a printer's error. They manipulated that table, but it doesn't matter, because the facts are in the paper.' *2019-04-09*

He was on a roll. 'Here's this guy [Rossouw] sitting next to me telling the UCT audience *that* we don't know how to control obesity, but he can't control his own obesity. I've lost 18 kilograms by changing from the diet that he advocates. I know exactly what causes obesity. He doesn't have a clue, and yet he's put up as an expert. It's astonishing!' An impish smile returned to his face. 'In my view, if you are not prepared to lecture on nutrition without your shirt on, then you shouldn't be talking about nutrition. If you can't solve your own problem, how can you possibly help others?' *2019-04-09 I lost around 23 kilograms.*

Stung by the intensity of his reaction, I lost my place in the notebook in which I had scribbled my questions. Flicking back the pages, I stumbled across a comment *that* Michael Vlismas had made about Noakes: 'Beyond reproach – his quest for truth and honesty is something *that* I've rarely experienced. He is determined to find the truth about a situation, irrespective of the cost to him. It's almost as if it's his life's mission.' *2019-04-09   2019-04-09   –To Daryl Ilbury is for Noakes*

It was clear that Noakes was passionate about his discovery, committed to getting it out there, and frustrated that his fellow academics seemed resistant to afford him the respect that he deserved. He obviously wanted them to listen and to even just think about what he was trying to say. Challenging convention is never easy, I thought, but when that convention is rooted in something as important as science, and especially medicine, and where principles are clouded by sensitivity and the welfare of patients is at stake, trying to shift mindsets must be not only physically demanding, but also emotionally shattering.

I closed my notebook, switched off the voice recorder to show that I was happy with what I had learnt, and we chatted for a while about sport and about how the book was going. Noakes asked me about the title. I admitted I hadn't given it much thought, but that these things normally came to me at some stage.

I thanked Noakes and we shook hands, agreeing to exchange further questions and notes if needed, and he ensured that I had copies of documents that I had requested. I then left the coolness of the Sports Science Institute of South Africa and stepped into the hot, brewery air. As I walked back to my car, I thought of the one question that I had asked of every one of those I had interviewed so far. As an opener, I had asked each of them to give me five words to describe Noakes. Ticking them off in my head, I found a remarkable degree of consensus: honest, loyal, passionate, and fearless but humble. There was another word that kept cropping up: quiet. Jake White spoke of Noakes having a 'quiet authority', Michael Vlismas about his 'quiet energy', and Lewis Pugh a 'quiet confidence'.

I sensed that somewhere among this collection of adjectives there was a title of a book, or at least a part thereof. Then I remembered how Lewis Pugh had answered that question about Noakes's character. I opened my notebook and quickly flicked through the pages until I found it. Circled and punctuated with a large exclamation mark were the words 'quiet maverick'. I thought it perfect, except for the fact that for over 40 years, Tim Noakes has been making a lot of noise.

See page 66.
2019-04-09

Chapter 6

Prometheus rejected:
Science in the media

Deep inside the hushed archives of the ivy-covered Jagger Library at the University of Cape Town sits the silent testimony to Noakes's rather vociferous relationship with the media. It awaits anyone wanting to dig deeper into an understanding of how Noakes has used the mainstream media over the past 40 years and how the media have portrayed him. I made an arrangement with Clive Kirkwood, who oversees the special collections and archives at UCT, to sit down with the collection and work my way through it. Kirkwood is the archetypal librarian – studious, softly spoken, somewhat protective towards his charges, but at the same time genuinely excited to share them with anyone who asks.

On the day in question he placed a large crate, piled to the top with thick A2-sized scrapbooks, in front of me. I promised him I would look after it. 'Oh, that's not everything,' he smiled, 'there's more.' He pointed to a nearby trolley heaving under a tower of boxes, each one of them filled with folders. On the floor next to it was yet another crate, similar to the one on the desk in front of me, also filled with scrapbooks. I did some counting: 11 files with magazine articles, 10 files full of clippings from popular science publications, eight files of clippings from mainstream publications, 32 scrapbooks of newspaper clippings, one oversized folder of laminated articles, and a box of audio-visual recordings in various formats. The collection covered the years 1974 to 2012. Noakes had been busy. I asked Kirkwood if this was typical for an academic. He shook his head. 'The Tim Noakes Papers as a whole comprises a large archival collection; there's a small number of collections of academics that are more voluminous, but none that have anywhere near as large a media-coverage component.'

The material is a combination of articles written by Noakes, letters he has penned to newspapers, articles written about him, and articles in which he has been mentioned. There are also copies of speeches he has made, a collection of programmes from awards dinners where he spoke or was guest of honour, and clippings from his early days as a rower at university. Of special interest to me, however, were the newspaper clippings – pre-online news coverage. I was interested to see any evidence of Noakes having been a maverick, and, if so, how the mainstream media then portrayed him.

Several things became clear. Firstly, the vast scope of issues around sport, health and nutrition over which Noakes expressed an expert opinion was impressive. This was evident not only in the range of topics on which he spoke, but also in the diversity of publications. He either wrote about, or was featured in articles about, running, athletics, rugby, cricket, swimming, triathlons, biathlons, the mental and physical stresses of sporting competition, political decisions around sport, heart attacks, obesity and nutrition, to mention just a few. His articles appeared in just about all the mainstream South African newspapers – English as well as Afrikaans – and in a number of overseas newspapers and magazines. And not only in sports sections in newspapers and in sports magazines such as *Sports Illustrated* and *SA Runner*;

I also found articles in women's magazines, such as *Fair Lady* and *Personality*.

Secondly, I was struck by the respect that the media seemed to have had for his opinion; there was almost a pride in his international stature as a scientist. He was always presented as a specialist, even when what he was saying was clearly rattling convention and public opinion. An example was his call for stricter safety regulations in rugby. Noakes was accused of 'softening' a game that was at the heart of the steely Afrikaner identity. At the centre of the controversy is a letter sent in 1987 by Dr Danie Craven, then president of the South African Rugby Board, to the Spinal Cord Injuries Centre at Conradie Hospital in Cape Town, requesting that they no longer use Noakes, claiming that he was 'biased' and that his work was 'to say the least, unscientific'.

Noakes's fight to get the South African Rugby Board to recognise the risk of spinal injuries in rugby continued for many years, often playing out in the media. One article from *The Argus* of 19 January 1991, headlined 'Sports war of words could end up in court', speaks of Noakes's opinions on rugby injuries 'earning the wrath of the South African Rugby Board', especially of a senior official, Pietman Retief. But then it immediately talks of Noakes as 'the proverbial prophet without honour in his own country' and refers to his 'international acclaim as an academic'.

In the article Noakes refers to the 'public attack' on him, by Retief, that was playing out in certain elements of the media, and which eventually swung against Retief, resulting in his resignation from the board. There were some jibes; I found a number of examples of when Noakes was accorded the title 'Professor Tim Noakes and the Mothers Brigade' for his continued 'vendetta against rugby', and letters from readers with recommendations that he keep science out of sport; but on the whole, there seemed to be support from sports writers who sensed that Noakes was

2019-04-09
Good to be
cynical.

onto something. There was, of course, another explanation for all the good press in the folders in front of me: Noakes only submitted articles that supported him. I made a note to ask him at our next interview.

2019-04-09

The third thing that was clear was that Noakes certainly had an eye for the camera. Amid all the articles were numerous pictures of him in the ubiquitous cheesy pose usually demanded by newspaper photographers: pretending to be running, holding a plastic heart while pretending to be running, kneeling with a stopwatch next to someone else pretending to be running, holding a stopwatch next to someone actually running on a treadmill while plugged into all sorts of apparatus, and holding various laboratory equipment while not running. I mention this because just about every scientist I have ever interviewed made a point of telling me that they didn't want to be photographed in any kind of cheesy pose. That such pictures of Noakes are aplenty either pays tribute to Noakes's willingness to take one for the team, or underlines a slavish desire to get his face in the papers.

Overall, though, wading through the media archives made me realise to what degree Noakes stands apart from other South African scientists when it comes to engaging with the media. This is something to which Marina Joubert is particularly attuned. Joubert is an award-winning science communicator and a science communication researcher at the Centre for Research on Evaluation, Science and Technology (CREST) at Stellenbosch University, near Cape Town. Her work focuses on research in the fields of science policy, scientometrics, evaluation, and science and technology studies. As such, Joubert has the ear of many of the country's scientists wanting to connect with non-scientists about their work. She tells of a time when she interviewed Noakes to write a story for the newsletter of the NRF. 'He told me then that if a week went by without a request from a journalist for a media interview, he would find a reason to call one of his many media contacts.' That may sound arrogant, but he certainly knows how the media works and values their role in getting his message out. He readily admitted to Joubert that his high public profile helped him attract top students, collaborators and research funding. But that came at a price, according to Joubert: 'Even then, some of his peers disapproved of his high media profile, but they could not fault him on academic credibility.'

For Joubert, Noakes is a typical high-profile scientist who doesn't shy away from controversy and notoriety, and thrives at the centre of attention, 'certainly an exception to the norms that govern conduct in the scientific community'. There are other scientists who fit this bill, just not South African. A term often bandied about to describe Noakes is 'celebrity scientist', and we'll find out later what he thinks about that. Joubert prefers 'visible scientist', the term suggested by Rae Goodell during the mid-1970s when she was working towards her doctoral thesis at Stanford University's Department of Communication. The work developed into a book called *The Visible Scientists*. Goodell interviewed 40 leading scientists to see why it was that the likes of Margaret Mead, Carl Sagan, B.F. Skinner, Linus Pauling and William Shockley caught the imagination of the American public. She went on to form the Massachusetts Institute of Technology's first science writing programme, and today, under the name Rae Simpson, she is a leading science writer.

Goodell qualified 'visible scientists' as those ready to break old rules of protocol in the scientific profession, question old ethics and defy the old standards of conduct. Writing in the January/February 1977 edition of *The Sciences*, she explained that what makes them 'visible' is their comfort in circumventing traditional channels for influencing policy – i.e. academia – by taking their message directly to the public. She says a visible scientist typically 'has a hot topic, is controversial, is articulate, has a colourful image, and has established a credible reputation'.

There's an interesting caveat that Goodell emphasised: most of the visible scientists are protected from possible establishment pushback because they enjoy 'academia's version of job security: tenure'. This seems to encourage visible scientists to often talk beyond just their science itself, to the implications and ramifications of it. 'They are mavericks, tilting with the establishment,' Goodell wrote. 'Consequently, they are often outsiders – even outcasts – in the scientific community. Their colleagues may view them almost as a pollution in the scientific community – sometimes irritating, sometimes hazardous. They cause consternation among science-watchers and policy-makers and concern that they will mislead the public when they speak outside their areas of expertise as they often do.' Consequently, and Joubert agrees, visible scientists are much discussed, but also idolised, cursed, applauded and ridiculed.

So is this the case with Noakes? I asked Joubert how accurately and fairly the media was presenting Noakes. She smiled with the resignation of someone well experienced in the not-so-subtle idiosyncrasies of the media. 'They're covering the issues and developments around Noakes as one would expect the media would – according to its own rules and criteria,' she said. She pointed out that Noakes uses traditional and social media to influence public opinion, and that now that he's in the public limelight and facing opposition, he has no choice but to keep playing by the media's rules: 'The way that the media reports about science never is – and probably never will be – scientifically accurate. Journalists write to please their editors and their audiences, not scientists. Consequently, inaccuracies and hype creep in. However, much of the sensationalism that journalists are often accused of may actually originate from scientists and research organisations themselves, who have a vested interest in attracting media attention to legitimise their work. And, as Noakes is well aware, controversy always makes news.'

At this point you may be wondering, if the media shapes your view of science, how can you expect to get a balanced perspective? There are specialists for this task, and they're inspired by the tale of Prometheus.

According to Greek mythology, Prometheus, a titan, forged mankind from clay. Knowing that in order to survive mankind needed fire, he lit a torch from the sun and brought it to Earth. Zeus considered the fire as stolen, and was so incensed that he punished Prometheus – an immortal – by having him chained to a rock, where a giant eagle tore at his liver every day, the deity version of being forced to listen to ABBA's 'Dancing Queen' over and over again. — Humor.

It's a myth imbued with themes of discovery, bravery and loyalty, which is why Prometheus's name is often embraced by popular science. But it's his action of bringing fire, and therefore knowledge, to mankind that is the reason why the analogy of Prometheus is often used by Professor George Claassen to describe the role of science journalists.

Claassen is the popular archetype of a senior academic: bespectacled, with tousled greying hair, and a subtle, endearing air of eccentricity. He also has an inextinguishable passion for science and science journalism. He has to – he presents the only course in science journalism in South Africa, at Stellenbosch University. Therefore, no accurate tale of science journalism in South Africa is possible without tapping into his research and opinion.

A former deputy editor of the leading Afrikaans daily *Die Burger*, Claassen started the course in 1995. At the time it was the first of its kind in Africa. Ask him about the Prometheus analogy, and he explains that in the early days of journalism, journalists were often compared to the mythical Greek hero. 'Unfortunately,' he says, 'in South African newsrooms, editors have replaced the basic fire of knowledge that journalists should bring to the people with the burning desire to feed the masses with information about celebrities and royalty, their sex lives, where they dined last night, and with whom.'

It's not a casual observation. Over the years Claassen has been driving research examining the levels of understanding of science among media consumers, journalists and editors. The situation, he says, is unhealthy.

'The South African media in various ways neglect reporting on scientific discoveries and developments; and when journalists do report on science, the quality of reporting is often open to criticism from the scientific community.' He quotes a report from 2004 which showed that less than 2 per cent of editorial space in the country's top publications was awarded to the topics of science and technology. And those were the good ol' days.

It's one of a number of studies in South Africa that has tapped into a tangle of cultures, tensions and failures; and a public simultaneously interested in, confused by and fearful of science.

South Africa has a sobering science literacy rate. A study by the Human Sciences Research Council found that of those who did go to school, 30 per cent never studied maths, 55 per cent never studied physical or chemical science, and half of them never studied biological science. Successive World Economic Forum Global Competitiveness Reports rank South Africa near the top in terms of the efficacy of corporate boards, the regulation of securities exchange, the protection of minority shareholders, the legal rights index, and the strength of auditing and reporting, but near the bottom in terms of maths (math) and science education at high school.

Failures in maths and science education impede the country's development. Katy Katopodis, group editor-in-chief of the independent news service Eyewitness News, points out that this is why it is politically very sensitive, often making headlines, especially when the matriculation results are announced. 'We can't talk about the shocking state of maths and science education in South Africa without talking about the fact that there doesn't seem to be the political will to address the state of education in this country,' she says.

The issue of education cuts deeply in a country that was socially and economically divided during apartheid, and where demonstrations by schoolchildren in 1976 sparked the Soweto uprisings that became the rallying cry for urgent political change. Today, education is seen as pivotal if the country is to reverse decades of poverty and economic imbalance. Issues around education have become touch-paper to the tinder-dry sentiment of frustration around overall government failure with regard to service delivery.

In late 2015, universities around the country ignited into violent protests spurred by demands for affordable and accessible tertiary education. The war cry #feesmustfall morphed into calls for the 'decolonisation' of curricula, faculty representation, even entire institutions. At one stage it entered the realm of the bizarre, with a demand that science itself be 'decolonised' and focus instead on more 'traditional' understandings and interpretations of science, such as the apparent capacity of witchdoctors to send bolts of lightning to strike people.

Superstition and a belief in spirits are endemic to traditional indigenous cultures and, as such, South Africans are prone to embrace what science journalists dismiss as pseudoscience. Most newspapers feature regular astrology columns, and any whiff of magic is carried quickly through communities willing to attach any measure of hope for a better life.

It's something that concerns scientists and science journalists alike. Claassen quotes a study of his where there was strong agreement by both journalists and scientists to the statement that 'the South African public is gullible about much science news, easily believing in miracle cures or solutions to difficult problems'.

Trying to 'sell' science to the South African media-consuming public also suffers from the issue of public priorities. The country battles extraordinarily high levels of violent crime, an issue that dominates the minds of most South Africans; it crosses all cultural, political and socio-economic divisions. With such powerful drama and emotional issues so prevalent in the lives of South Africans, it's easy to understand why science battles to find a foothold in newsrooms.

Katy Katopodis admits that crime and politics dominate the South African news landscape, leaving little space for science stories: 'There's never a dull or "no-news" day. Every day is a busy news day with brutal crime and political dramas.' She says that science, if featured, usually provides some measure of balance, and often finds itself as an 'and finally' story. 'You can't bombard the listener with crime and politics 24/7. We have to let the listener breathe a bit and know that there is some good news going on – it's that balance of light and shade, and science often fits the bill.'

If science is tagged on to the end of radio news stories, it's virtually non-existent in regular programming. Katopodis admits that on the talk stations serviced by Eyewitness News, science stories are often buried in general programming. 'In a three-hour talk show, the first couple of hours will focus on current news events, and a science story or feature, if carried, will appear towards the end. In our defence, because of the nature of our newsroom, it's difficult to prioritise science stories.'

If South Africa had a champion of science in the media it was Christina Scott, who was killed in a car accident on 31 October 2011. A tireless campaigner for science journalism, Christina was the science editor at the SABC for both radio and television between 1994 and 2004, before becoming a regular science writer for the *Mail & Guardian*, one of the few remaining investigative titles. At the time of her death, she was also the host of the only science programme on SABC's flagship English national radio station SAfm, *Science Matters*. I asked Lynn Smit, former secretary of the South African Science Journalists' Association and a close friend of Scott, the reason for her popularity. Smit replied that it was Scott's ability to connect with scientists and help them really share what they were doing. 'She also made science fun.'

The death of Christina Scott left the station, and indeed the entire SABC, with a challenge in terms of how to cover science. But where some see only challenges, others see opportunity. Paul McNally is a journalist and author and the brains behind *The Science Inside*, a programme that launched in February 2014 on Voice of Wits, a radio station that broadcasts from the journalism department at the University of the Witwatersrand. I met McNally and his team shortly before their first broadcast. They had sent me a copy of their pilot show and asked me for feedback and input. I was immediately struck by the passion and focus of the team. McNally's impetus for the project was the very inertia that others voiced around getting science on radio. 'The idea for *The Science Inside* was based around the resistance from the people around me – including journalists – to produce a science show,' McNally said. There was plenty of money for the project; it was an appetite for science that seemed lacking. 'The problem wasn't around the will of the department to fund, but an exaggerated shrug from people in my circle that science is not news.'

But McNally is not one for 'no', and he had an idea for making science 'news': finding the science *within* the news. He was to tell me a couple of years into the project: 'We would take protests, for example, and create science stories around that "news" topic. This could be, say, the psychology of crowds or how a stun grenade works. In my mind a "failed" show was one simply around SKA [the Square Kilometre Array radio telescope] and a successful show was one where we managed to work an SKA story into a show about a politician getting stabbed.' The result was a series of programmes that took their cue from current events: the science of water restrictions during a drought that struck the city, of viticulture at a time of a popular wine festival, of elections when they came around, and of that ever-present pestilence – crime.

Identifying science in everyday life is easy; a key challenge for McNally to covering that science on radio was getting scientists prepared to talk about it. So he turned to Anina Mumm, a trained biochemist and journalist with an eye for a story and empathy for the reticence of scientists to engage with the media. 'My role was primarily to find experts and to hold their hand through the process,' Mumm told me. 'I reached out to them, discussed potential interview angles with them, asked them to help us identify important issues, prepped them for live interviews and helped them communicate technical info in a more accessible way.'

I asked both McNally and Mumm about the challenges of working with scientists, and about the impact of Tim Noakes on science in the media. McNally suggested what he thought was a problem in covering science – the reluctance to be interrogative – and pointed to a show they did on Noakes as an example. 'If you don't come out in the positive, then I think listeners are often left wondering why they were told the story in the first place. I feel that this need for science journalism to be positive, to fill the space of an "uplifting piece" on the news cycle, allows people like Noakes to go by without being properly shaken. I think we were probably too kind to him.' *[handwritten: that]* *[handwritten margin: 2019-04-09]*

Mumm remembered that programme: 'We asked researchers involved in the studies around the sugar tax to speak to us about their work and about the sugar tax in relation to Noakes, and they refused, because, I think, they found it too controversial to link their work to Noakes in any way.'

Both McNally and Mumm have since moved on. Mumm became a science communication and digital media specialist at ScienceLink, South Africa's first digital science communication start-up, and chairperson and volunteer editor at SciBraai, a not-for-profit organisation dedicated to science journalism, science communication and outreach in South Africa. If there's a future for science in the South African media, it lies in the hands of people like Mumm.

If there's a more pressing reason for the coverage of science in the South African media, it's this: the very health of the nation is at stake. According to the World Health Organization, almost 54 per cent of South African adults are overweight, and 26.8 per cent are considered obese. Other surveys show slightly different results, but they all agree that South Africans are getting bigger; in 'media-speak', obesity is reaching epidemic proportions. This is a major concern, because obesity invites numerous health problems, such as hypertension and cardiovascular diseases; respiratory problems, such as asthma; musculoskeletal diseases, such as arthritis, high cholesterol, diabetes and some forms of cancer. It seems now is a good time for scientists to speak out about South Africans' eating habits. Therein lies a problem. *[handwritten margin: 2019-04-09]* *[handwritten margin: almost 80.8% of people are overweight or obese.]* *[handwritten margin: 2019-04-09]* *[handwritten margin: 2019-04-09]* *[handwritten: Cholesterol does not really matter for heart disease?]*

Getting scientists to speak to the media is very much a 'rock-and-a-hard-place-meets-chicken-and-egg' scenario. Most scientists I have interviewed distrust the media, complaining *[handwritten: whom]* *[handwritten margin: 2019-04-09]* that when they have spoken to the media, they have either been misquoted, or their work misrepresented. In a discipline that demands accuracy, and where character and credibility are key, this is especially problematic. Many scientists have told me that they risk 'character assassination' if they are either highly profiled or misquoted in the media.

On the other side of the coin, for reasons presented earlier, the media are generally ambivalent towards science, their assumption being that their audiences don't have the appetite for it. As a result, I joke that my role as a freelance science journalist working through news editors requires taking something that someone doesn't want to share, and sharing it with someone who isn't interested, using the help of someone not particularly helpful.

South Africans are not alone in losing science coverage in the news; it's a global issue sparked by shifts in media consumption patterns and the costs of production, especially after the 2008 global economic downturn. The warning shots were fired in early December 2008, when CNN cut its entire science, technology and environment news staff. CNN spokesperson Barbara Levin explained at the time that they were going to 'integrate environmental, science and technology reporting into the general editorial structure rather than have a stand-alone unit'. That's corporate spin for 'axe'.

Other news organisations around the world followed CNN, and the coverage of science has largely been taken from specialists and handed to mainstream journalists, often with little interest in the topic. In South Africa, things are particularly bleak. Sarah Wild, a multi-award-winning science journalist, has a more brutal appraisal: 'There is very little science journalism. There are only a handful of beat journalists who cover science, and it's usually science within health, the environment and education.'

Wild also taps into that old common misperception: 'Science

is often considered "too difficult" or "too technical", and so is marginalised by news editors. In South Africa, many of the people who are news editors now were political reporters in the 1980s, which means that their focus is politics.' A glance at most of the stories dominating South African news media would support that, as would the current affairs sections of local bookstores. Then, of course, there's that issue of money. 'Given the shrinking resources in newsrooms,' says Wild, 'science is considered a "nice to have"; it is definitely not a focus of any newsroom in this country.'

It is rare nowadays to find a science desk in a major newsroom. There are exceptions; in 2011 I was assigned to the science desk at the *Financial Times*, one of the world's biggest news titles. But even there it comprised only two journalists – Clive Cookson and Andrew Jack – and a lot of their news consisted of covering events in the pharmaceutical industry. The coverage of science in the news media now is the responsibility of a tenacious band of freelance science journalists, still burning the Promethean flame.

Such journalists are only part of the corps of people in the media shaping your understanding of the science at the heart of this book: human nutrition. There are others, and here I must explain the difference between a science journalist, a science writer and a science communicator. Because their roles can overlap, it makes things a little complicated, but there is an important difference, especially when it comes to the truth in what you read, see and hear: a science journalist is a qualified journalist, whereas a science writer or communicator doesn't have to be a journalist. An important distinction is that journalists are schooled in the rigours and discipline of journalistic ethics and integrity. I say that with a heavy heart, because there seems increasingly less evidence of this in what is emerging from the mainstream media nowadays. Tabloids spew out the ethical equivalent of clubbing baby seals in a school playground.

Journalists are therefore expected to follow a strict code of behaviour based on their awareness of, and sensitivity to, legal issues around such things as defamation, malicious falsehood, confidentiality, privacy and copyright, and ethical issues such as reporting on children, representing victims of crime, balance of evidence, protecting sources and breach of confidence. Essentially, journalists should display responsibility and accountability in the collection and dissemination of media content. They should report the facts, with an eye for balance and fairness. Now ask yourself if that's what you get on social media. ⌐ *incisive comment.*

A science writer is someone who tells the story of science, employing a more narrative style. In my opinion, some of the best science writers are scientists who know how to tell a story. This means abandoning the rigidity of academic writing and reaching for their inner poet, lyricist or storyteller. Examples include astrophysicist Carl Sagan, evolutionary biologist Richard Dawkins and theoretical physicist Stephen Hawking.

Science writers can also simply be writers with a Zen for the beauty and mystery of science. Carl Zimmer is an excellent example. He writes for the *New York Times*, *Discover* magazine and *National Geographic*, and is responsible for one of the best opening lines in popular science writing: 'It is as astonishing as it is sad to watch a ladybug turn into a zombie.' It's from an article in *National Geographic* about wasps with a penchant for laying their eggs in living insects. The story is titled 'Mindsuckers', and I urge you to look it up; unless of course you scare easily.

Generally speaking, these writers tell their stories with an eye, and ear, for the lay audience; hence the term 'popular' science. But the format remains the same: it is generally longer than something written by a science journalist, with a freer-flowing, more relaxed style, and embraces the tools of creative writing. Science journalists can also be science writers; they simply adapt their writing style accordingly.

The role of science communicators is in their title: to com- 2019-04-09 municate a concept in science. They may employ writing as part of their brief, but essentially they are tasked with a purpose to convey clarity on a point about science. This means that 'science 2019-04-09 communicator' is a title that can be given to a staff member of a science museum, someone writing for a biomedical company that produces science equipment, or a spokesperson for a research institution. But it can also be employed to describe a PR officer for, say, a dietitians' organisation whose job entails producing media releases. So science communication is not averse to the occasional spin.

Closer to accuracy, a science communicator can also be a scientist with a knack for popularising their field; Neil deGrasse Tyson is a case in point, as is Tim Noakes.

The importance, especially in South Africa, of encouraging scientists like Noakes to communicate their work is the impetus of Marina Joubert's research into the 'science of science communication', and it is shedding light on the political nature of science and the intricacies of communicating science in diverse social settings. What Joubert and her colleagues at CREST have learnt is that knowing science doesn't necessarily equate to *loving* science. This seems counter-intuitive, and, if correct, threatens to overturn traditional models of science communication.

'In fact,' says Joubert, 'more information about science may make people more worried about science. People respond to scientific information in complex ways, and their responses are shaped by their own background, experiences and views. There- whom fore, understanding and respecting the audience you are trying 2019-04-09 to engage is an absolute prerequisite for effective engagement.'

There's that concept that many scientists find so bohemian: 'engaging' with the public. However, Joubert and her team propose an even more demanding intervention to heal the ills of a public ignorance of, and suspicion towards, science: 'meaningful communication'. Joubert explains: 'It involves mutually beneficial dialogue between scientists and communities – listening to people's concerns and expectations – rather than a one-way, top-down flow of factual information.' This can be done face to face, or on social media. She then whips out the 'r' word that boils the blood of many science academics: 'relevance', the belief that science should connect with people's everyday lives. According to Joubert, science communication is therefore not about promoting science, but rather about embedding science in society and allowing people to participate in science. The very idea is anathema to hard-core scientists, and, it's fair to say, is also something most people would rather do without.

This discordant interface of science and society is something Toby Murcott struggles with every day. Murcott is a scientist by training, now a multi-award-winning science writer, journalist and broadcaster, and a former lecturer in science journalism at City, University of London. He is also a teacher in science communication, so he wears all of the above hats with the word 'Science!' on them. He agrees that the roles of science journalist, writer and communicator often overlap: 'A science journalist, like a science communicator, must make the topic of their research or investigation clear to the audience; point out to them that this is how it may impact their life.'

He is quick to clarify the key differences, though: 'A science communicator is essentially an advocate for science, whereas at all times a science journalist is an intelligent and friendly critic.' Would it be fair to say science communication is PR while science journalism is investigating under the skin of science? Murcott is a little more diplomatic: 'In a nutshell, a communicator represents their client, a journalist the audience.'

He then explains some of the realities of a journalist in a disrupted media environment: 'Any journalist today is being asked to produce more for less. Ten years ago a journalist may have been a straight print journalist, whereas now they would be expected to contribute content across multiple platforms and formats, such as podcasts or video, and for print and online; and if it's online, regular updates, with all the necessary adaptive criteria, such as encouraging click-throughs and page views. What was a clearer role 10 to 15 years ago is now blurred. There's a need to make a story go further, which means inevitably there is less time to go and gather original stories.' So where does the content come from? He sighs. 'As a science journalist, you are more reliant on press releases and content that comes to you from other sources than securing your own content.' The end result spells bad news for those wanting to dig around in possible bad science. 'There is less time and money to do more investigative journalism,' he laments.

It is from the public relations industry that science journalism in South Africa is facing one of its biggest challenges. As seasoned science journalists are cut from their desks, PR teams of research organisations and science-based companies are enjoying a more enthusiastic, and unquestioning, embracing of their press releases. It's not uncommon to see swathes of recurrent copy – and a common voice – in different news outlets covering the latest research. The result is the impression of a singularly accurate narrative.

For those science journalists still trying to cover science accurately, one of the biggest challenges they face is sidestepping those press releases to get face-to-face time with scientists, and developing relationships with such sources. The relationship between scientist and journalist is a cautious one, with scientists usually protective of their research and journalists inclined by instinct and profession to probe at it.

For Lynn Smit, the problem lies to a degree with the attitude of those conducting the research. 'It's an academia thing, not just science. They sometimes have an arrogant attitude that they are the holders of this great knowledge and that everyone else is going to misquote them.' She says that scientists often want to see the stories before they go to print, and a lot of the younger journalists don't realise that they are under no obligation to send their work to scientists to be checked.

However, without the proper context from a scientist and a robust examination of their research, says George Claassen, what often happens is that highly complex research findings are reduced to misleading headlines and reports that present deductions that are either exaggerated or blatantly wrong. Add in a snappily crafted but carefully skewed press release, and a rapidly advancing deadline, and the temptation by inexperienced journalists to copy and paste without examination and investigation is strong. This isn't helped by a sub-editor who knows that hyping a headline will earn it online traction, click-throughs and engagement on social media. The result: a twisting of the truth that is embraced as fact.

With all this in mind, I ask Murcott about how nutrition is being covered in the media, and point to the media uproar around Tim Noakes. Murcott has a renowned impish character that comes to the fore when explaining key components in the covering of science, and it takes this opportunity to step into the spotlight. 'Whatever you read in the media about nutrition, the first thing you've got to remember is that it's almost certainly not true.' He pauses for effect, sensing my shock. 'What you're reading is a very small piece of a very large jigsaw, and all the pieces add up to an overall view of a particular topic.' Content is king, context is King Kong.

So what should a media consumer look out for in a nutrition story? What questions should they ask of it? Murcott slips on his science-journalist lecturer's hat: 'The first thing to look for is, does the journalist provide any context – any backstory – and any opposing views? Is there any nod to a bigger picture? If not, then bells should start ringing – this could be "churnalism", something simply churned out from a press release, with no critical examination by a good science journalist.' He wags a finger. 'And, of course, it may not be true; it might be part of a bigger truth, and if you treat it as a black-or-white truth, that's not going to work.'

Of course, up until this point, references to the truth in 'the media' and the role of science journalists, writers and communicators in influencing the perceptions of media consumers have focused on only one sector – what is now called 'mainstream media' – newspapers, magazines, radio and TV. Importantly, these organisations covering news employ the services of journalists who are supposed to observe strict regulations and codes of practice, especially around issues of accuracy and fairness.

The internet and the explosion of social media has changed this media environment, wresting the legacy of media from mainstream. Media consumers are now also content producers; they are 'prosumers'. This has dramatic implications: should you tell Betty Sue about the wonders of your new diet, that's a private conversation. If you write the same story on Facebook, it makes you part of the media, and, therefore, theoretically, subject to the same rules and conditions. Some pundits call this the 'democratisation of the media', but in effect it's created a disrupted media landscape where accuracy and fairness have fallen by the wayside in the grapple for the attention of the media consumer, and where rules no longer seem to apply.

So how influential is social media in how we make sense of the world around us? In May 2016, the Pew Research Center, a US non-partisan 'fact tank', published a report that found that a majority of American adults (62 per cent) get news on social media. According to the data, 66 per cent of Facebook users and 59 per cent of Twitter users get their news from their respective sites. This is slightly above the global average, and that makes sense, given the fact that the US often sets the trend in media consumption. Research published in 2016 by the Reuters Institute for the Study of Journalism found that, across 26 countries, an average of 51 per cent of people access news through social media on their smartphones. It's fair to assume that as the spread of smartphone usage increases and the cost of data decreases, that number will only go up.

If forming an accurate understanding of science demands critical thinking, having more open access to information should be a good thing. But when it comes to social media, two things conspire to curb our critical thinking: personal bias and the machinations of the matrix into which we are plugged.

It's tempting to believe that we are insightful and open to new ideas, but that's not entirely true. Daniel Kahneman is a specialist in the field of the psychology of judgement and decision-making; he is also a winner of the Nobel Prize in Economic Sciences. In his bestselling book *Thinking, Fast and Slow* he explains that every day we are confronted by a mind-boggling amount of complex sensory data, in reality far too much for our brain to break down and analyse every time. Instead, the brain groups data together into clusters of identified and assumed associations. This developed repository of learnt responses is what Kahneman refers to as System 1 thinking. It is impulsive and emotional. It's what steers us to immediately look towards the sound of an explosion to assess the possibility of danger. But it's also sensitive to short-circuiting: the screech of a train as it pulls into a station can quickly evoke memories of your childhood, spinning on a squealing playground roundabout.

System 2 thinking is slower and more methodical. It handles 2019-04-10 the learning of new skills, and steers logical reasoning and in-depth analysis. It's more effortful and demands more attention. It's why you often get hungry when you are studying. There is less emotional association in System 2 thinking, unless, like a researcher, you get a kick out of correctly connecting seemingly disparate dots.

If we were to apply Kahneman's classification to the con-sumption of media, watching a dancing kitten on YouTube taps into System 1 thinking, whereas analysing a scientific paper about nutrition, where the content is largely new, draws on System 2 thinking.

But there's another component to social media that's import-ant when it comes to engaging with science, and it's what makes it 'social'. Qualification for content generation and dissemination is not gauged by accuracy, but by self-image management and the opinions of others within a social grouping. Unlike a journalist 2019-04-10 clinically approaching a topic and publishing a balanced article in mainstream media with a focus on factuality, users of social media are steered more by emotion and are less likely to differ on opinion around an issue if it risks their alienation. For some of the same reasons, humans make bad subjects for research – they yearn for social acceptance, they are susceptible to peer pressure and they are inclined to acquiesce to authority – they are easily influenced on social media. As a result, personal bias can take hold.

There's another major flaw in accessing and sharing news on social media that entrenches this bias and contributes to the polarising of opinions: the matrix. As much as you'd like to believe that 2019-04-10 you can pick and choose the news on Facebook, the reality is that it's already chosen for you. At the heart of the selection of news content for Facebook users are the algorithms designed to draw the user to content that is aligned with their interests and opinions. According to Will Oremus, senior technology writer at *Slate* magazine, the secret algorithm – and it's continually changing – scans everything you've posted, everything your friends have posted and linked to, everything you've clicked on, and every Facebook page you've liked, and processes it. No one outside a select few at Facebook's Menlo Park head office in California knows for sure how this is done. That's scary. Juxtapose that with the fact that the staff at any mainstream media outlet are usually known and accessible, so there's always responsibility and accountability when it comes to their generating media content.

Think about that for a minute: instead of the critical eye of an experienced journalist schooled in the rigours of investigation, and expected to balance the weight of differing evidence and opinions on a matter in which they are specialists, the flow of information arriving on your screen is censored by a mathematical algorithm.

But there's another problem: if the algorithm is generating content based on what you *like* and who you follow, it obviates potential exposure to content that may *challenge* your preconceptions. The net result – and if you're a Facebook user you may have noticed this – is that you find seemingly overwhelming support for your opinions; so you begin to believe that you're right in the way you think, and that any challenge to your opinion must be wrong. The result: an increasing risk of polarising sentiment and the development of communities constructed around a particular opinion; consumers become either for or against an issue in the media.

Twitter works in a similar way. When you check your timeline, you may notice that the tweets at the top are not necessarily the most recent. It's Twitter's 'Show me the best tweets first' feature.

It's like the 'While you were away' feature that was introduced in 2015, and is driven by a similar algorithm that determines what it thinks is most relevant to you. According to Twitter product manager Michelle Haq, it was designed to address the so-called FOMO effect: the human fear of missing out. The result is similar to that of the Facebook news feed: a collection of stories that will probably enforce your bias – that what you believe around issues such as politics, religion and human nutrition is right, and if anyone says otherwise they must be wrong. So let's say you click on a link to an article that's in favour of a specific diet or eating lifestyle: chances are you will come across more links to more articles supporting it.

The overall impact is that instead of accessing diverse and detailed contextualised content around an issue – through properly mediated platforms – and applying rigorous analysis, with the associated effortful System 2 thinking, more people today are connected, through social media, to the emotional, quasi-instinctive entrenchment of preconceived biases more associated with System 1 thinking. The result is the development of what's called a 'filter bubble' – a cognitive isolation where what's received reaffirms pre-existing bias.

This can encourage the separation of media consumers on social media into opposing 'camps' around those few science issues of seemingly any relevance, and especially so for those even fewer issues about which those consumers are passionate. This builds tension, and leads to the exchange of verbal slings and arrows without the restraints of journalistic ethics and integrity, or any fear of the consequences of unfettered opinion.

This is why social media is so reactive. To ignite a social media firestorm, all it takes is for a maverick scientist with a high media profile and a penchant for tweaking a nerve to step up and say something, especially about an issue as divisive as what you put in your mouth.

Chapter 7

Human nutrition:
It's not a soundbite, people!

Regardless of what you gather from the media, there's no binary thinking in science; no either this or that. This is a cause for confusion when we are comfortable with the idea that there are two possible options for any stance. For example: you're either for or against abortion; you're either conservative or liberal; someone's either innocent or guilty, rich or poor, or, the classic South African construct, black or white.

The problem with binary categorisation is that it polarises. People become split into two tribes; and, given the human inclination to favour emotion over rational judgement, such camps see the other as villains and bristle with distrust and suspicion. All it takes is a spark to create all-out war. Sectarian violence based on self-created and arguably pathetic religious, cultural, ethnic or tribal polarisations are the brutal embodiment of such binary categorisation.

Make no mistake, binary *relationships* do exist in science, but they don't suffer the human perceptive classification of a cause for war. In astronomy, a binary star is a star system composed of two stars; in biology, binary fission is the splitting of a single-celled

organism into two daughter cells; and in chemistry, a binary com-
pound is one that contains two different elements, for example
H_2O. Importantly, however, in these examples the split is not con-
frontational; both units co-exist in some measure of harmony.

Of course the most familiar example of a harmonious binary
relationship in science is found coursing through the arteries
of information technology: data in the form of strings of binary
digits, the smallest unit of data used in a normal computer and
having a value of either 0 or 1. However, even that difference isn't
so cut and dried. Scaling down into the elusive arena of quantum
computing, a qubit (quantum bit) can exist in a supposition of
both states, meaning it can represent a 0 and a 1 simultaneously.
So, even in the cold, calculating world of physics, there's a case
for ambivalence.

And yet something akin to a cleaving has occurred in our
modern understanding of human nutrition, and it dates back to
an unfortunate event on 23 September 1955. President Dwight
D. Eisenhower was enjoying a game of golf at the Cherry Hills
Country Club golf course, just outside Denver. At the eighth hole
he started to complain about feelings of indigestion. At 02:00
the next morning he awoke with chest pains, and his attending
physician, Major General Howard Snyder, administered mor-
phine, believing erroneously that the president had indigestion.
It wasn't until 12 hours later that an electrocardiogram (ECG)
showed that Eisenhower was, in fact, experiencing an acute myo-
cardial infarction; the president of the United States was having
a heart attack. He was rushed to hospital, where he stayed for six
weeks before being released with a warning to keep a lid on his
infamous temper and cut down on his four-pack-a-day smoking
habit.

Two things happened while Eisenhower was in hospital that
are important for our story. Firstly, he insisted that the American

public be kept fully informed of his condition. This wasn't Trump-esque bloated self-importance; instead, it was a more selfless understanding that his health was of national concern. Eisenhower was a war hero, the former Supreme Allied Commander in Europe, and a popular president. At the time of his heart attack he commanded an approval rating of 79 per cent, and as news broke of his condition, the Dow Jones dived by over 6 per cent, losing $14 billion in value by the end of the day. It was the worst single day for markets since the attack on Pearl Harbor. Eisenhower knew that rumours about his health were dangerous for the US economy. He was also aware that he was not alone – American men seemed to be suffering more and more heart attacks. At that time, estimations were that about 800 Americans per 100 000 suffered from heart disease. There seemed to be a national condition that demanded dramatic intervention.

The second thing that happened is connected to the first: Eisenhower was put in touch with a man who seemed to have an answer to this condition. That man was Ancel Keys, a University of Minnesota–based pathologist, and his work had captured the attention of Eisenhower's personal physician, Dr Paul Dudley White. Interestingly, Keys's and Eisenhower's paths had already crossed: it was Keys who had developed the famed K-rations first used in the US military during the Second World War – the K stood for Keys.

That, in a way, captures the character of Ancel Keys. He was self-confident to the point of arrogance, believing that it was the responsibility of other scientists to prove his research wrong, rather than his to question himself. He wasn't a medical practitioner, but he did qualify with a PhD in physiology from Cambridge University in England in 1936, and developed a special interest researching possible links between diet and disease. He was famously combative and intolerant of those who had the audacity to question him. But he was also charismatic and knew the value of surrounding himself with powerful people. He had a comfort with publicity and knew how to work the media. At a point when questions were being asked about the health of the nation, Keys considered it his duty to take charge.

Keys told White that Eisenhower's condition stemmed from his smoking and his love of fatty foods. For example, we know that on the day of his 'indigestion', Eisenhower had consumed a breakfast of sausage, bacon and hotcakes, and for lunch a large hamburger with raw onions. Keys said that if Eisenhower wanted to live a long life with a healthier heart, he had to change his diet by cutting down on fat. Keys thus became the champion of what was to become the 'diet-heart hypothesis' – the belief that fat in food was linked to the build-up of cholesterol 'plaque' in the arteries, thereby contributing to an increased risk of heart attack and stroke.

Cholesterol is an important part of the cell membranes in the body; it's a waxy-like substance that regulates what goes in and out of cells. However, if cholesterol was linked directly to the build-up of atherosclerotic plaque, it made sense to Keys, and to those he could influence, that reducing a build-up of cholesterol could be as simple as reducing its intake in saturated fats – the naturally occurring fats found in animal foods such as meat, milk, butter and eggs, as well as certain plants such as coconut and palm oil. It certainly sounded logical.

Not everyone agreed. Across the Atlantic Ocean, Britain's leading nutritionist, John Yudkin, had a different theory: that heart disease was linked to the consumption of sugar, not fat. Importantly, he had the research to back up his theory. Yudkin was, in character, the complete antithesis of Keys. He was quiet, reserved and intensely scholarly, with little predilection for self-promotion. He did a PhD in biochemistry at Cambridge, before completing his MD in 1938, also at Cambridge, researching intermediary carbohydrate metabolism; so he would have been at Cambridge at the same time as Keys. At the time of Eisenhower's heart attack, Yudkin was a professor at Queen Elizabeth College in London and had been instrumental in developing a department responsible for cutting-edge research into nutrition.

Yudkin's research also echoed that of other European nutritionists, especially those in Germany, Italy and Austria, who were champions of endocrinology – the study of hormones, their effect on the human body and the diseases that result, such as hyperthyroidism and diabetes. For them, the link between saturated fat in food and the development of atherosclerotic plaque was too simplistic. They believed that the intricacies of the human digestive system held other secrets to heart disease, and if there was a key to unlocking it, it was sugar.

There was some logic to this, too. Refined sugar is a relatively new addition to the human palate and so, from an evolutionary perspective, the human digestive system is only just trying to make sense of it. Saturated fats from animal products, however, are an old friend of the human gut.

It's perhaps a good idea at this juncture to try to make sense of just how intricate and complicated the process of human digestion is, because it is critical to what has been termed the 'low-carbohydrate, high-fat (or LCHF) debate'. This requires a quick lesson in biochemistry, which you're more than welcome to skim through if you know your calcium from your iron and your triglycerides from your cholesterol. However, a refresher lesson won't hurt anyone.

It's easy to think back to the periodic table in your science classroom, rattle off the better-known chemicals and point to the inanimate objects around you as artefacts (artefacts) of those chemicals. But the same is true for us; and if you want to feel special, know that key chemicals in your body – hydrogen, oxygen, carbon, nitrogen, calcium and phosphorus – were all coughed up by collapsing stars and supernova explosions. As Carl Sagan famously said, 'The nitrogen in our DNA, the calcium in our teeth, the iron in our blood, the carbon in our apple pies were made in the interiors of collapsing stars. We are made of starstuff.' *2019-04-10*

According to the Second Law of Thermodynamics, all closed systems – and you could be considered a closed system – have an increasing tendency towards disorder. Reversing this requires the continual input of energy. However, the human body is not like a steam engine; it is a living organism made of chemicals. To prevent disorder, it therefore needs to process – like a factory – the chemicals in food to build and maintain its intricate network of biological structures and procedures. To remain optimally operational, it attempts to keep everything in a state of metabolic balance – homeostasis – especially with regard to temperature, fluid volume, calcium levels, acidity and glucose concentration. Evolution over hundreds of thousands of years has got the system down to be pretty effective.

Essentially, once food is swallowed and enters the digestive system, enzymes from the pancreas help break up the food into *2019-04-10* its different molecular components. These are then absorbed and reassembled into other molecules and compounds that are necessary for the healthy growth and reconstruction of the various components of the body, such as muscles, bone, skin and hair. The chemical composition of the human body is highly complex, but essentially the main components of human cells are lipids (fat-like molecules that are insoluble in water), proteins and carbohydrates, and there needs to be a balance of all three from the food that we eat to ensure healthy cell structure, function *2019-04-10* and energy provision.

There's a key component to fats that makes their role in our bodies particularly complicated: their diversity – there's no such thing as a single 'fat', whether it be in the food we eat or the lipids in our body. Just as there are saturated fats, there are other fats that occur naturally – such as those in certain plants like avocados, certain seeds like sunflower seeds and pumpkin seeds, and nuts – and that are called unsaturated fats. Saturated fats are normally solid at room temperature; unsaturated fats are liquid. Generally speaking, though, because they are naturally occurring, saturated and unsaturated fats can both be considered healthy, or part of 'real foods'.

Trouble can arise when certain fats are changed for the manufacturing of processed foods and so-called fast foods. In a process called hydrogenation, natural liquid vegetable oils are heated in the presence of hydrogen gas and a catalyst. When these vegetable oils are partially hydrogenated, their structure changes to the point at which they can withstand heat, which makes them suitable for frying fast food. They are then called trans fats, and have become a mainstay in restaurants and the processed-food industry – for frying, baked goods and processed snack foods. Trans fats may be convenient, but generally speaking, because they don't occur naturally, they can be considered unhealthy.

Once these different fats are processed in the body, they are converted to organic lipid molecules, the most important of which – at least for the purposes of this story – are cholesterol and triglycerides. Where these two differ is in their design and purpose. Cholesterol is made in the liver and in part by the wall of the small intestine, and is designed to help construct things, like cells and certain hormones. Triglycerides, which are also made in the liver, are designed to be broken down. They are the storage vessels for unused calories – to provide your body with energy when needed. Between building cells and providing those cells with energy, cholesterol and triglycerides are among the most important lipids in the body. They are, however, rather bothersome. They don't dissolve in blood, which makes them difficult to transport from the organs that make them to the cells where they are actually needed. So they hitch a ride inside a clump of certain proteins, and the resultant particles are a marriage of lipids and proteins called lipoproteins.

These particles float around in the blood to get to where they need to do their work. Problems occur, however, if, instead of rushing off to work, they gang up like disaffected youth along the walls of the arteries, restricting blood flow and damaging the walls, or break off in clumps and head off in search of trouble in the heart or brain. The lipoproteins that do this are called low-density lipoproteins (or LDL). Other lipoproteins with a higher density have less of a tendency to attach themselves to arterial walls, preferring instead to barrel along in the blood to where they're supposed to go. This is why high-density lipoproteins (or HDLs) are often referred to as 'good cholesterol', and their lighter-density cousins, 'bad cholesterol'. Either way, the logical thing should be to give lipids work to do so that they use the energy they store, i.e. exercise.

Again, if only it were that simple. Although it's easy to think that the processing of food only takes place in the gut, it actually requires a seamless connection with many major organs in the body. The beauty of the system is in the checks and balances, in the regulatory role of certain organs, particularly the liver (the more cholesterol in the food you eat, the less your liver produces). But other organs play a key role, too, and one of the most important is the pancreas. It's not only part of the digestive system, excreting enzymes into the gastrointestinal tract to help break down the proteins, lipids and carbohydrates in food; it is also part of the endocrine system, secreting two essential hormones directly into the blood: glucagon and insulin. Hormones are special chemicals that trigger a response in the body: glucagon

2019-04-10

tells the body to boost its blood sugar levels, and insulin to reduce them. These two hormones work in tandem, like yin and yang, to maintain a balanced supply of energy to the cells. Insulin production really kicks in to lower blood sugar when you eat carbohydrates, which, compared to fats, release their potential energy easily.

Because all the organs of the human body interact with one another to try to maintain homeostasis, if one organ is over-worked and doesn't stay up to speed, the whole process can become obstructed, and even shut down. So it makes sense that if we can simply understand more fully how a human factory works, then it should be relatively easy to determine what is the best combination of food going in to get the most effective operation and, therefore, the best output.

Not so fast. This is when things get positively labyrinthine. Just as any factory requires a programme that regulates operations, so do humans. This is determined by our DNA, the programming code in every cell and our resultant genetic definition. Any fault in the programming will result in the incorrect distribution of chemicals and compounds – not enough here, too much there – resulting in physiological imperfections such as male-pattern baldness and dwarfism. Although humans naturally share a broadly defining programming code, there are a myriad refining differences that are responsible for diversity within the species, with the required different chemical demands; e.g. melanin for skin and hair colour, or calcium for characteristic skeletal struc-ture such as height and shape of the head. Accordingly, this helps account for the differences in diet found around the world, lactose tolerance being an example.

End of the biochemistry lesson; now back to Ancel Keys.

2019-04-10

Given the chemical complexity of the human body and the unlimited diversity within the human species, it seems rather ridiculous that any government could determine what everyone should eat. And yet this is what Keys had in mind in the years following Eisenhower's heart attack. He started wielding his considerable charisma and domineering character to entrench himself within institutions that would provide opportunity to influence health-care policy. Two of those institutions held particular sway: the National Institutes of Health (the US national medical research equivalent of South Africa's NRF) and the American Heart Association (AHA), of which Eisenhower's personal physician, Paul Dudley White, was a founder. Keys worked his way onto the boards of both. From this base he encouraged the allocation of funding to researchers who supported his diet-heart hypothesis, and found every opportunity to canonise what would become one of the most controversial studies in human nutrition: the Seven Countries Study.

From 1958 to 1964, Keys led a team of researchers who conducted observational research and data analysis of 12 770 middle-aged men in seven countries: the US, Greece, Yugoslavia, Finland, Japan, Italy and the Netherlands. The team, with the help of scientists in the host countries, collected extensive data on the eating and lifestyle habits of these men, as well as their general health, as measured using specific biomarkers such as serum cholesterol and ECGs. Keys then correlated that data with evidence of heart disease and any related outcomes, such as death. The idea was to plot the fat intake in each country against the number of deaths related to heart disease in that country, and then assess any correlation.

To the casual observer this all sounds pretty impressive, and it must be emphasised that at the time this was cutting-edge research. In the late 1950s there was no such thing as 'big science', and in the words of Henry Blackburn, one of the study's chief coordinators, 'there was neither precedent nor support for a properly organised, rigorous, centrally directed, adequately funded, multi-centre undertaking'. But having now been exposed to some of the restrictions of scientific research and the opportunities for wayward analysis, you've probably heard some bells ringing. The first, of course, is that the Seven Countries Study only examined men, mainly middle-aged. Reasons given at the time were the invasiveness of the field examinations and that heart attacks seemed more rare among women. So that's half the human population already excluded.

Secondly, the obvious question: How were the seven countries selected? That is one of the most controversial components of the study, with many accusations over the years of selection bias – that Keys cherry-picked countries he already knew had both high levels of fat in their diet and high incidences of heart disease. Indeed, had he selected to study, say, the Inuit of Canada, he would've found a diet high in fat and a people with relatively few incidences of heart disease. South Africa was one of the countries originally identified by Keys, but abandoned because of perceived challenges obtaining data, and, in the rather disconcerting opine of Keys, 'the fact that no one seemed to be interested in imitating the ways of the Bantu'.

Thirdly, and critically, the study should have been interpretatively capped by that unwritten credo of scientific research: correlation doesn't necessarily mean causation. However, before the Seven Countries Study even started, Keys had already published – in no fewer than 20 papers in top scientific journals – his claims that total cholesterol in blood could be reduced by cutting back on saturated fats. He now needed evidence to back it up.

Other issues have since arisen that have limited the scope and impact of the Seven Countries Study, and these have been acknowledged by no less than Henry Blackburn himself. In a retrospective of the study available on the website of the University of Minnesota School of Public Health, Blackburn lists some of the limitations. These include the selection of samples in different geographic areas in part for reasons of convenience, and the technical challenges of conducting surveys across cultures by national teams, often working under difficult field conditions.

Another of the study's chief coordinators, Alessandro Menotti, has gone further. Many years after the conclusion of the study, he re-examined the data and found that the food that most closely correlated with deaths from heart disease was, in fact, sugar, not saturated fats. This had been suggested to Keys a number of times during the roll-out of the study, but summarily rejected.

In essence, the Seven Countries Study was a bold, ambitious and exciting observational study, and it provided insight into a *possible* correlation between the lifestyles of *carefully selected, gender- and age-specific subjects* and heart disease. As such, it should have been part of a much broader series of studies and, importantly, the inspiration for randomised controlled trials to get a bigger, more accurate picture. Instead, it was heralded by Keys as the academic authority to discharge dictates of what all people in the US should and shouldn't eat, and started the foundation for what some have called a nutritional house of cards that would show the signs of strain on closer investigation. Enter Nina Teicholz.

Within journalism, special regard is accorded to the investigative journalist; they're akin to a mix of detective, hacker, surgeon, terrier and storyteller – a journalist's journalist. While most journalists attempt to report on the facts with an eye on the editor tapping their watch, investigative journalists eschew such trifles as deadlines, concentrating rather on getting to the bottom of the story, no matter how long it takes. The Academy Award–winning film *Spotlight* gave us a rare glimpse into the impact that such dedication to investigative journalism can have; in that case, the

understatement. (?)
2019-04-10

exposure of systemic sexual abuse by Catholic priests in Boston. Investigative journalists live the credo of journalism's ABC: accept nothing, believe no one, check everything; and they know that if you want the real story, you often have to follow the money. For all their stature within journalism, investigative journalists usually operate under the radar, and for them the kick is connecting the dots, not the glare of publicity. They often avoid the limelight, preferring to probe within the shadows of subterfuge. Truth be told, investigative journalists can be a strange bunch, science investigative journalists possibly even more so.

To that end, Nina Teicholz is something of an aberration. Attractive, arguably glamorous, but quietly spoken, Teicholz doesn't immediately come across as intimidating, but she has emerged as a formidable challenge to nutrition convention and the institutional corpus behind it. She has, to her merit, a quiet composure and an unremitting drive to uncover all the facts, follow all the leads and arrive at the big picture within which the current nutritional guidelines have taken shape. Teicholz is an independent science investigative journalist and the author of one of the most detailed, meticulous and uncompromising exposés of the corrupt mash of science, politics and big business: *The Big Fat Surprise*. So important was the book to a detailed understanding of nutrition that when it was published, the *American Journal of Clinical Nutrition*, a premier journal in the US, described it as a 'historical treatise on scientific belief versus evidence'. *The Economist* declared it the top science book of 2014.

For Teicholz, a turning point in human nutrition came when, after Eisenhower's heart attack, the American Heart Association, flush with cash following successful fund-raising efforts initiated by food and consumer goods giant Procter & Gamble, formed a nutrition committee with the hope of securing some measure of certainty about the causality of heart disease. Various hypotheses emerged, including obesity, vitamin B deficiency, lack of exercise, blood pressure and stress. Interestingly, any link between saturated fat and heart disease was largely dismissed. This was because successive studies worldwide up until that point had failed to find any.

That changed when, in 1961, Keys, through his influence on the AHA nutrition committee, managed to secure a turnaround in opinion to the point that the committee issued a report claiming that the best scientific evidence available suggested that 'Americans could reduce their risk of attacks and strokes by cutting the saturated fat and cholesterol in their diets'. It also recommended the substitution of saturated fats with unsaturated fats such as corn or soybean oil. That must have made Procter & Gamble happy.

According to Teicholz, the 1961 AHA report was the first official statement by a national group anywhere in the world recommending that a diet low in saturated fats be employed to prevent heart disease: 'It was Keys's hypothesis in a nutshell.' For context, she goes on to explain that the influence of the AHA on the subject of heart disease was – and still is – unparalleled, and that the dietary guidelines published by that committee 'have been the gold standard of nutritional advice'. So impactful was the report that Ancel Keys made the cover of *TIME* magazine in 1961, a major event for anyone, let alone a scientist.

Keys never seemed to consider that he was wrong. He wasn't interested in testing his hypothesis, only in confirming it, and would, with the might of the AHA and the NIH behind him, often publicly attack any researcher who challenged him. Amid the characteristically reserved and quantifying academic community, Keys was better at playing the political game, or as Teicholz prefers to say, 'the blood sport of nutrition science'.

As his influence over nutrition policy developed, Keys became emboldened, and took aim at any study from leading researchers worldwide that challenged his hypothesis. And there were many, such as research by the World Health Organization, published in 1964, which examined the diets of men virtually free of heart disease, and concluded that any attempt to find a link between the two was unreliable. There were also individual researchers who would become thorns in the side of Keys's diet-heart hypothesis.

One was Dr Edward H. Ahrens, or as he preferred to be called, Pete Ahrens. He was a respected clinical investigator based at Rockefeller University in New York, and a specialist in lipid metabolism (how the body processes fats). Like Keys, he was interested in any possible link between diet and atherosclerosis. But his research differed from Keys's in two main respects. Firstly, he was always firmly academic and resisted making public health recommendations in the absence of clear experimental proof. Secondly, his focus was not on cholesterol – the so-called building block of cells – but triglycerides, those lipids designed to be broken down to provide the body with energy when needed.

Ahrens's research discovered that high triglyceride levels were far more common than high cholesterol in patients with coronary disease, and hypothesised that triglycerides were a better indicator of a propensity for heart disease. But that wasn't what threatened to upset Keys's diet-heart hypothesis. Because high triglycerides were found in people with diabetes – who also had a higher risk of heart disease – the two diseases had a common contributory cause, namely excessive weight gain. Ahrens believed that a possible agency was an inability to properly process carbohydrates. Because a diet low in fat is usually offset by being high in carbohydrates, if Ahrens was right, a low-fat diet could make things worse, especially for people with any genetic predisposition towards diabetes.

In many ways Pete Ahrens was, like John Yudkin, an ideological counterpoint to Ancel Keys; and because of his commitment to a focus on academics rather than policy, he was overshadowed by Keys, who captured centre stage in steering discussions around human nutrition.

With few academics, especially in the US, willing to publicly challenge Keys and his colleagues at the AHA and the NIH, funding was funnelled to those researchers who were likely to support the diet-heart hypothesis. Many of these studies were epidemiological – they examined diets against heart disease within populations and made a *retrospective analysis* looking for associations. Few were proper clinical studies because of the obvious challenges of limiting extraneous variables when applying some measure of nutrition intervention; ask any parent who's tried to get their child to eat spinach.

At this juncture you may be thinking that all this is fascinating, but what does what happened half a century ago in the US have to do with me here, and now? The answer lies in what could be described as scientific hegemony. The US spends more than any other country on scientific research and development. For the 2015–2016 financial year, the US federal government budgeted $135.4 billion for research and development; granted, the bulk of it on defence (more bang for your buck). Add in private investment in R&D, which is approximately twice as much as what the federal government spends, and you can understand why the country is a technological powerhouse.

Where the US really flexes its muscle, though, is in *academic output* and influence. In terms of the number of academic papers published, and the number published in the top 10 per cent most cited, the US is clearly dominant. Citation is important, because it's a measure of the impact – or the academic footprint – of the research. Whereas Test batsmen in cricket are ranked according to batting averages, scientists move up and down the rankings according to what is known as their h-index (or Hirsch index), a

2019-04-10

2019-04-10

2019-04-10
My papers were not important.

2019-04-10

125

mathematical measurement of academic productivity and impact: the higher the h-index, the greater the academic impact. It's very technical and not without its critics, but a figure often used for context is the following: every year the US National Academy of Sciences inducts members in recognition of their distinguished and continuing achievements in original research; membership is a widely accepted mark of excellence in science and is considered one of the highest honours a scientist can receive. In the year the h-index was first suggested – 2005 – the median h-index among the 36 new inductees into the National Academy of Sciences in biological and biomedical sciences was a highly admirable 57. In case you're wondering, Tim Noakes's h-index in 2016 was far higher: 71.

The SCImago Journal & Country Rank is a publicly available portal that ranks science journals and country scientific indicators based on leading bibliographic databases. Between 1996 and 2015, the US published 9 360 233 academic documents, more than twice as many as second-ranked China; but, importantly, whereas those documents received 202 750 565 citations, an average of just under 22 citations per document, Chinese documents commanded an average of just under six citations. As a matter of interest, in the ranking of 239 countries in terms of academic output, South Africa sits at 34. Not too shabby.

It's fair to say that in terms of global academic impact, the US swings the biggest sledgehammer, and this is important when considering international academic-backed public policy.

In 1977, the US Senate Select Committee on Nutrition and Human Needs, influenced by the work of Ancel Keys, issued dietary goals for the US that included an increase in carbohydrate consumption to about 60 per cent of energy intake, and a reduction in overall fat intake to 30 per cent, of which saturated fat should constitute only a third. Since then, every five years from

1980, the official dietary guidelines for Americans have been published by the Department of Health and Human Services and the Department of Agriculture, and every year saturated fats have been the whipping boy.

Of course, the focus of these guidelines is not the American home-cooked meal. The entire US convenience-food industry – the R&D, operational, logistical and marketing costs big food companies incur in the design, manufacture, distribution and advertising of their products – hinges on the public accepting that what they buy is based on the veracity of the nutritional guidelines that support it. This affects everything from food production to food labelling and public feeding programmes, used by about a quarter of the US population. What if those guidelines were overturned? What if the guidelines suddenly switched and said 'actually, we're wrong about the whole low-fat thing'? What would be the implications? And this isn't just a US issue; given the global reach of so many US convenience-food brands, what ends up in a microwave in Soweto may not be all that different to what goes into one in Seattle.

To this end, it is in the interests of food companies that the nutritional guidelines don't change; that there are no shock events that would demand a complete reassessment of every component of their product lines. And that's why one of the first things a science journalist does when they examine any research into nutrition is look to see who funds it. Every scientist has to include on any paper they publish the details of any possible conflicts of interest. This includes the name of any funder that could benefit from publication of the outcome. Scientists and their funders know this, so a lot of research in nutrition is funded through organisations and lobby groups, which in turn receive funding from large food companies – often unfairly grouped together under the inimical sobriquet 'Big Food'. There's nothing wrong with this; big food companies need the latest nutritional research, so they help by investing in it. The problem comes when there are strings attached to such industry-funded science.

It's tempting to think of industry scientists, their lobby groups and so-called Big Food as akin to an axis of evil, an apocalyptic ensemble of Dr Evil–like villains continually scheming in underground bunkers, pinkie fingers to their lips, cackling with ungodly malice as they steer the consumer into an early grave. In fact, that wouldn't make sense. To paraphrase another movie character, Nick Naylor in *Thank You for Smoking*, how on earth would Big Food profit from the loss of its consumers? It's in their best interests to keep their consumers alive and eating their products.

I thought, given the depth and breadth of her investigation, Nina Teicholz would be the best person to try to present a snapshot of any connivance that shapes the way we eat. So I contacted her in New York. She quickly poured cold water on any suggestion that Big Food was pulling all the strings. 'I don't blame the food industry entirely for our food guidelines going wrong. The ultimate gatekeepers who sit on expert panels are academic scientists; they're supposed to weed out bad industry-funded science and influence from the good science.' So scientists are at fault?

'This story is really about a failure of science. It's about scientists who fell in love with their own hypothesis about what constitutes a healthy diet, couldn't let go of it, selected evidence to support it, and ignored or suppressed evidence that contradicted it.' She then went on to explain how the food industry responds to the guidelines. 'I have interviewed hundreds of food-industry executives; the guidelines are like a straitjacket to them. They respond to the guidelines faithfully. If they're told, "make foods that are low in fat", they make foods that are low in fat. They just want to say their foods are healthy and in line with the guidelines. That "healthy stamp" is decided by scientists.'

I couldn't believe that with its wealth, influence and invest- 2019-04-10
ment, the food industry was just tagging along. Teicholz agreed,
and pointed to all the vested interests in affirming the nutritional
status quo. 'These include not only the food industry, but university scientists who have been endorsing and promoting these
guidelines, and who sit on all the expert panels, the AHA who
first recommended the diet, and let's not forget all the pharmaceutical companies that support all the medical associations and
who sell the products that these sick people need.' She paused and 2019-04-10
then pointed out the forgotten elephant in the room: 'The US Very important.
government would be liable if the guidelines are found to be the
cause of obesity and diabetes.' For Teicholz it makes sense that 2019-04-10
all these vested interests cannot acknowledge that the current
nutritional guidelines might be causing epidemic diseases; and
that for economic, professional and institutional interests, they
cannot back out of this failed hypothesis.

'All of these forces coming together are like a bulwark against
change,' she explained. Furthermore, according to Teicholz, they
are not only resisting change, but also effectively suppressing
those encouraging it. 'There is a network of mainly scientists, 2019-04-10
possibly fuelled by industry money, from Harvard, Yale, NYU
[New York University] and the CSPI [Center for the Science of
Public Interest] in Washington, D.C., that takes an active part
in taking down those of us who are trying to expose the flaws in
the science.'

Embracing change to correct such flaws in our knowledge is
paramount in science; this is what separates it from dogma. The
continued awareness that what we know from scientific enquiry
is provisional and subject to adaptation, change, even overhaul, is
supposed to be built into the logical construct of every scientist;
so the suggestion by Teicholz, that narrowly defined yet broad-
reaching prescriptions about human nutrition are embedded

within science, was unsettling. That other forces were at work to ensure this was upsetting. The integrity of my field of interest as a journalist and writer seemed broken.

The alternative was that Teicholz was irrational, overly suspicious, borderline paranoid. And yet evidence of such suppression of the challenging of convention is on public record. In October 2015, the *British Medical Journal* (*BMJ*), one of the world's oldest and most respected medical journals, published an investigative article by Teicholz titled 'The scientific report guiding the US dietary guidelines: Is it scientific?' The article was solicited by the editors of the *BMJ*, and fact-checked and peer-reviewed per *BMJ* procedures.

The CSPI immediately posted a rapid response, alleging that the article was 'error-laden'. Teicholz responded, providing further evidence to back up her claims. However, instead of continuing an open debate, a group within the US scientific community decided it should be shut down, permanently. On 5 November, the CSPI issued a letter demanding that the *BMJ* retract the article – a very serious course of action for any journal.

However, as a result of the brutal pushback, the article spilled from the venerated halls of academia into the roughcast avenues of mainstream media, something that perhaps the CSPI hadn't intended. Signatories to the letter started distancing themselves from its contents, and hyperbole around the supposed inaccuracy of the article was downgraded from 'error-laden' to a specific number: 11. The *BMJ* fact-checked, *again*, the supposed errors, and published its findings that they were either insignificant or purely semantic and had no bearing whatsoever on the veracity of the article. Teicholz remained transparent throughout the whole process, publishing everything on her blog The Big Fat Surprise, together with links to all the evidence. She also uncovered that the signatories of the CSPI letter included all the members of the 2015

Dietary Guidelines for Americans committee, all the living authors of the Seven Countries Study, scientists involved in the American Heart Association and others, including environmental scientists, management consultants and graduate students, a majority of whom appeared in a somewhat reproving light in her book.

Ian Leslie, an investigative journalist for *The Guardian*, managed to track down and interview many of those who had signed the letter, and discovered intriguing discrepancies in their objections: 'They were happy to condemn the article in general terms, but when I asked them to name just one of the supposed errors in it, not one of them was able to. One admitted he had not read it. Another told me she had signed the letter because the *BMJ* should not have published an article that was not peer-reviewed [even though it was].'

Final vindication for Teicholz came in December 2016, when the *BMJ* issued a statement saying that, after further critical evaluation, they stood by her article and would not retract it. For the layperson this may sound like an incidental academic triumph, but in reality the consequences are profound, especially for Noakes. It meant Teicholz's 10-year investigation, which uncovered that the scientific foundations of the US Dietary Guidelines – as well as those around the world – were faulty and prejudiced, had been accepted into the corpus of international scientific knowledge. The *BMJ* statement went on to say that 'criticisms of methods used by the [US Dietary] Guidelines Committee are within the realm of scientific debate, and merit further investigation of the composition of the committee'.

Teicholz could be forgiven for being bitter, even mistrustful, but there's little evidence of it in her temperament. She seems to relish the fight, finding solace amid the mountain of evidence she has amassed over the years, as well as the sense that she might actually make a difference in helping to reverse chronic disease.

Others, though, have shown less sustenance in their taste for battle. Teicholz rattled off a number of names of health professionals who have suffered the slings and arrows of what could be called the 'nutrition establishment'. Two are worth mentioning, both Australian.

In August 2016, after a two-year investigation by the Australian Health Practitioner Regulation Agency (AHPRA), Gary Fettke, a leading orthopaedic surgeon based in Launceston, Tasmania, was told to stop giving nutrition advice. Fettke alleges that a dietitian based at the hospital where he worked complained to the AHPRA that he was telling patients, mainly those with diabetic foot complications, to adjust their diet to incorporate more fat and fewer carbohydrates, and to cut processed food and sugar intake as recommended by the World Health Organization.

It's important at this stage to clarify the difference between a dietitian and a nutritionist; the two terms will start popping up from now on. The regulatory specifics differ from country to country, but in essence the difference is one of academic rigour and clinical authority. Whereas 'nutrition' is a broad term applied to (healthy) human eating habits and lifestyle, a 'diet' is a specified nutrition regime for a specific reason or occasion. This means that dietitians are authorised to provide clinical therapeutic intervention to patients and are allowed to work with doctors, whereas nutritionists are not. To qualify as a dietitian therefore demands a higher, more exacting level of academic study, usually a bachelor's or master's degree in dietetics, and all dietitians have to be registered with their country's respective health professions body. Having said that, it is possible for a nutritionist to be a senior academic; John Yudkin was a case in point. It means that their field of research is human nutrition; however, importantly, they are still not qualified to dispense clinical dietary advice (unless they are also a qualified dietitian).

132

Back to Gary Fettke. He may have been based in Tasmania, but he was no backwater doctor. He was well known and respected for founding the Nutrition for Life clinics, designed to help guide patients to develop a better understanding of nutrition, especially around diabetes. According to Jason Fung, a leading Canadian specialist in kidney disorders, Fettke founded the clinics after becoming disillusioned with amputating diabetics' limbs while he believed that the disease could be easily managed with proper nutrition. Fung says that he had the exact same epiphany a few years ago: 'I was sick and tired of putting diabetics on dialysis when the entire debacle is preventable with a proper understanding of nutrition.'

The resultant AHPRA investigation into Fettke backfired slightly when it resulted in a government senate inquiry into the medical complaints process in Australia. Fettke gave evidence that he had experienced 'systemic bullying and harassment in the public hospital system' and 'a prolonged and vexatious AHPRA investigation'. He also spoke of 'a sustained defamatory campaign posted on a social media hate page that led to cyber bullying' of him, his wife, staff and friends.

If Fettke's experience was ruthless, that of Jennifer Elliott was brutal. Elliott was a registered dietitian based in New South Wales with 30 years' experience. For most of that time she implemented the established nutritional guidelines, including with her own family. For two of her three children it seemed to work, but one of them – her middle daughter – was seemingly always sickly and had a predisposition for putting on weight. By the time she entered her teens, she was, in Elliott's own words, 'borderline obese'. After a recommendation by a GP who had a similar situation with one of her own children, Elliott had her daughter tested for insulin resistance. The test came back positive. It showed all the symptoms of insulin resistance: high levels of triglycerides, elevated blood glucose levels, weight gain around the midriff, low levels of HDLs, and high blood pressure. In her search for a solution, Elliott discovered the link between cutting back on carbohydrates and a normalisation of the metabolic balance in others with a similar condition. She adjusted her daughter's diet accordingly, and her health dramatically improved.

Elliott kept up the research and started encouraging patients who were diabetic, insulin resistant or pre-diabetic to reduce their intake of carbohydrates and increase their intake of fat. In April 2011 she published a book titled *Baby Boomers, Bellies & Blood Sugars: How to lose inches, lower blood sugars and get your energy and life back!*

She did further research, working with GPs in her area who would refer to her any patients displaying all the symptoms of insulin resistance, and developed not only more evidence to challenge the current nutritional guidelines, but also growing support for her nutritional advice. Pushback eventually came in July 2014, when another dietitian lodged a complaint against Elliott with the Dietitians Association of Australia (DAA). Things weren't helped when, in October, Elliott published a paper in the journal *Food and Nutrition Sciences* titled 'Flaws, fallacies and facts: Reviewing the early history of the lipid and diet-heart hypotheses'. In essence, the paper echoed the evidence presented by Nina Teicholz and the confidence among a growing number of dietitians, nutritionists and scientists, including Tim Noakes, that the diet-heart hypothesis was so flawed that it shouldn't be used as the basis of diet recommendations.

In May 2015, the DAA deregistered Elliott, making her unable to work as a registered dietitian. The DAA failed to provide a detailed reason for their action. It certainly wasn't because she flouted nutritional guidelines for diabetics. Far from it. According to Franziska Spritzler, another Australian-accredited dietitian, now practising in the US and specialising in treating diabetics, 'Australia looks to the US, specifically the American Diabetes Association (ADA), as a trusted source of evidence-based information on diabetes management, and in the past the DAA have stated that they endorse the ADA guidelines for use by dietitians in Australia.'

She points specifically to a 2013 position paper 'Nutrition therapy recommendations for the management of adults with diabetes', which states, 'Evidence suggests that there is not an ideal percentage of calories from carbohydrate, protein, and fat for all people with diabetes; therefore, macronutrient distribution should be based on individualised assessment of current eating patterns, preferences, and metabolic goals. A variety of eating patterns have been shown modestly effective in managing diabetes including Mediterranean-style, Dietary Approaches to Stop Hypertension (DASH) style, plant-based, lower-fat, and lower-carbohydrate patterns.'

If the stories of both Fettke and Elliott sound familiar, it's because they suggest a pattern. I said to Nina Teicholz that it gave the impression that it was perhaps bigger than just Tim Noakes. She laughed with the wisdom of someone entrusted with the obvious, 'I *know* this is bigger than just Tim Noakes.'

Chapter 8

The trial

After chatting with Nina Teicholz, Tim Noakes's seemingly unscientific behaviour over the years started to make sense. In the years that followed my first interview with him in 2012, every time our paths crossed, we'd catch up and compare notes, and I would invariably comment on how he still had traction in the media – a major achievement for any science story. Each time he seemed to vacillate between being upbeat and frustrated, and this was reflected in the tone of his language.

On one occasion, on 5 August 2014, Noakes presented a talk at the Sci-Bono Discovery Centre in downtown Johannesburg as part of its National Science Week celebrations. I had been invited to introduce him and facilitate a question-and-answer session afterwards. As is usual at a Tim Noakes talk, the audience boasted passionate supporters, easily identifiable by the well-thumbed Noakes books clutched close to their chests, their enthusiastic nodding at the appropriate moments, and the echoes of adulation in their eyes. But these weren't adoring fans, they were people – mostly middle-aged – to whom Noakes was something of a saviour. They each had a story about how they had been on chronic medication for crippling life-threatening illnesses, but since changing their diet had cast aside their pills to walk unaided, with a renewed spring in their step.

Such adulation can be unhealthy for a personality, and make no mistake, Tim Noakes is a personality. It can poison humility and strip away meekness, and embolden a belief in invincibility. It's why much of my career as a broadcaster was spent tackling pop stars and politicians puffed up by a sense of self-importance.

As I listened to Noakes on this occasion, I suspected that he had befallen the curse. He remained firm on the line that for people like him, who were insulin resistant, a diet that was low in sugar-releasing carbohydrates and high in energy-supplying fats was the best course of nutritional action, and that the growing scientific evidence supported this. However, his talk and his answers to the questions afterwards were punctured by seemingly unscientific outbursts. There were lots of anecdotes, and as any scientist should know, the plural of anecdote is not data; but I ascribed this to his skill at communicating science and connecting with the audience. But there were also the repeated claims that powerful forces were attempting to protect what was akin to dogma, and that pharmaceutical companies made a profit from sick people who could otherwise get healthy simply by changing their diet.

I had tried to corroborate the seemingly wild things that he was saying with the seasoned academic that/whom I knew him to be. Because of the demands of peer review, scientists are renowned for their careful, qualified phrasing when answering questions, but the Professor Tim Noakes addressing the nodding audience was perfectly comfortable making what seemed to be wild accusations. Looking back on the notes that I made that day, I can see where I scribbled the word 'paranoid?' and circled it.

Afterwards I caught up with Noakes and challenged him, saying that I had found it quite uncomfortable listening to him talking about conspiracies to silence him. He smiled and said, 'But, Daryl, it's true; trust me, it'll soon all come out.' I was unaware at that stage that he knew an official complaint had been made against him.

The title of this chapter is "The trial."

In the years that followed, Noakes lost little momentum. He seemed to pop up anywhere to talk about his research, and that of others, which showed that a simple change in an eating lifestyle could have a dramatic effect on people with metabolic syndrome – that so-called cluster of conditions including high blood pressure and sugar levels, excess body fat around the waist, and abnormal cholesterol or triglyceride levels, which, together, can increase the risk of heart disease, stroke and diabetes. But most of all he became very vocal on social media, especially Twitter. If academic science has a publishing nemesis, it is Twitter. Substantive scientific knowledge grows from detailed intellectual academic discussion in peer-review journals, by known persons and accompanied by data and further detailed evidence. Twitter, however, is accessible to anyone, embraces anonymity and allows unsupported claims, limited to 140 characters or less. It therefore acts as an energy ramp for that ethereal source of popular reasoning, usually prefaced with 'you know what they say'.

This is why, when I teach scientists how to communicate their research, there is a noticeable reluctance to embrace social media. Younger scientists seem more open to the idea, but generally there's a disinclination to engage in a media space they see as frivolous, even dangerous. For them, it's a place for pop stars to share pics of their new shoes, attention-seeking politicians to peddle their idle thoughts, frustrated journalists to keep their opinions alive, and where people called @dogfart69 can wield the social fidelity that should only be accorded to philosophers. For scientists, if publishing had an axis of intellectual integrity, scientific journals would be at one end, Twitter at the other.

Although there's a merit of truth in all of this, what is unavoidable is that many leading scientists do use Twitter, especially those who see the value in communicating their research outside of the confines of academia and engaging directly with people about it.

Nevertheless, when Noakes fired off his first tweet, in April 2012, according to many scientists, he would have been turning his back on the exclusivity of academia and further embracing popularism. For others, it would have posed something of a threat. Given Noakes's popularity, his academic seniority and the unfettered reach of social media, his opinions on diet and lifestyle would have unlimited reach and immeasurable impact.

However, there's a flipside: social media also acts as a leveller, dishing out brutal rebuke if collectively warranted. Say something ridiculous, and it'll earn instant and continuous retaliation. It's why Twitter is a never-ending battleground of wills that can separate opinion into binary constructs, and the belief, when it comes to science, that things are either right or wrong. When it comes to something so complex as human biochemistry and nutrition, the resultant tension is virtually tangible, and sentiment sometimes borderline feral.

Why is this? Why is the matter of what we eat a source of such bitter disputation? If food simply serves the function of providing energy for our bodies, why should we be bothered with issues of aesthetics? The answer lies in our emotional connection with food: it is intimately intertwined with issues of social identification and self-awareness. Foods are anchor points in religious and cultural identities; for example, the eating, or not, of pork, beef, milk and shellfish. Meals are the centrepieces of family ceremonies, social discourse and intimate encounters; we 'get together for a braai', 'meet for coffee', 'do business over lunch' or 'have a romantic dinner'. But more than that, what we consume is connected with our self-image. It is part of the regime that defines us and tells others who we are; whether or not we eat free-range meat or meat at all, if we dine on sushi and champagne, or

burgers and beer. We are also socially catalogued by the brands that
we consume and where we consume them. But importantly, we
are told that what we eat is linked to how we look. Magazine
covers boast Photoshopped models and recipes to help you look
that good, and social media feeds off this fascination with body
image: '8 food swaps that will flatten your belly in a week', 'The
best diets for slimming the legs', '26 foods that will melt love
handles', and so on. These are genuine claims – Google them.

The importance of food is also captured in our media consumption. Walk into any leading bookstore and you will probably
find that the section or shelves dedicated to 'Food and Cooking'
will outsize any other; your local Sunday newspaper will no
doubt have a section dedicated to all things food; pop stars and
Hollywood actors are quick to endorse their latest weird diets,
which their slavish fans suck up; food-bloggers command page
views that mainstream news titles could only dream of; and there
are popular TV channels dedicated entirely to food and cooking.

Into this turgid culture of food and identity stepped Tim
Noakes on 5 February 2014, when he replied to a question posted
two days earlier on Twitter, addressed to him and Sally-Ann
Creed, a nutritional therapist (and co-author with Noakes of
The Real Meal Revolution). It was from a breastfeeding mother,
Pippa Leenstra: 'Is LCHF eating ok for breastfeeding mums?
Worried about all the dairy + cauliflower = wind for babies??'
Noakes's reply was the following: 'Baby doesn't eat the dairy and
cauliflower. Just very healthy high fat breast milk. Key is to ween
[*sic*] baby onto LCHF.'

It's neither an offensive tweet by any stretch of the imagination, nor does it fall foul of any media law – it's not libellous
and there's no encouragement of harm to others. People could
disagree with him and had a voice to do so; that's the point of
social media: it is a platform for public discussion. And people

did disagree, quite vocally, and there were others who supported his advice, equally vocally. Importantly, the question demanded a public, not private, response, which the person asking the question was free to accept or reject. And, as a medical doctor, Noakes didn't cross any ethical boundaries in replying on a public platform. He didn't publish any confidential patient information or dispense a diagnosis for a specific patient without seeing that patient; he simply provided generalised nutritional advice based on scientific evidence. Breast milk is high in fat, and there is scientific evidence to support the benefits of an LCHF diet. There is also evidence to the contrary, but, as we've realised, that's science for you. The secret in making sense of science is context, and this is where it clashes with social media.

The character limitation of Twitter is one of its selling points; it demands concise expression, a sub-editor's dream. It also means that tweets can be short on context, unless accompanied by click-through links to supporting evidence. Therefore tweets can be open to interpretation. However, this misses the main point of the brevity of Twitter messages: they are designed to encourage debate. Whether Noakes should have said 'Key is to wean *a* baby ...' as opposed to 'Key is to wean baby ...' is a matter for retrospective semantic debate. The fact is that he provided a broad opinion on a public platform as a scientist and researcher of human nutrition.

Importantly, in her original tweet, to which Noakes replied, Pippa Leenstra never referred to herself or her baby. She spoke of 'breastfeeding mums'. She was doing the media equivalent of asking a question in a town hall where the discussion was around LCHF. At that moment, Leenstra was a media consumer of medical or health information.

Not everyone saw it that way. One of those was Claire Julsing-Strydom, who at that time was president of the Association for

Dietetics in South Africa (ADSA), the professional organisation for the country's registered dietitians. Julsing-Strydom's reaction was to register a complaint with the Health Professions Council of South Africa. It was a decision that would effectively threaten to destroy Noakes's career, and make Julsing-Strydom the focus of a social media witch-hunt.

According to its website, the HPCSA provides the public with the right to request an investigation of any registered health practitioner whom they believe has acted unethically or caused harm. The site includes a downloadable form and an email address for Legal Med, the department within the HPCSA that handles complaints. To make sure that no health professional is a victim of a truculent member of the public with a hefty doctor's bill in one hand and an axe to grind in the other, there is a due process of investigation and assessment before any measure of disciplinary action is followed. Only the most serious cases demand a professional-conduct committee hearing, which is what Tim Noakes would be called before.

As I said at the beginning of this book, I am not going to go into the trial in detail; instead, I will focus on the following: the complaint, the charge that resulted, two key components in the case against Noakes, and the unexpected outcome of the hearing. The main focus will be on how this was all covered in the media.

By now you know that whereas content is king, context is King Kong, and in this case the context behind the complaint makes for interesting reading, for two reasons: firstly, it shows that Noakes's tweet was judged in isolation, and, secondly, it suggests that the complaint may not have been thought through.

What most people may not know is that directly after Noakes's reply on Twitter to Pippa Leenstra, someone else entered the discussion: Marlene Ellmer, a paediatric dietitian and someone well known to Julsing-Strydom. Ellmer tweeted the following:

'Pippa, as a paeds dietician I strongly advise against LCHF for breastfeeding mothers.' Leenstra replied by posing the following question to both Noakes and Ellmer: 'Okay, but what I eat comes through into my milk. Is that not problematic for baby and their winds at newborn stage?' Ellmer responded by tweeting another message with her email address, encouraging Leenstra to contact her directly. Noakes didn't do this, which is important to note, as we shall soon see. Leenstra tweeted to Ellmer that she would contact her, and after the discussion played out further with various people providing input, Leenstra tweeted: 'Thanks, but I will go with the dietician's recommendation.' This she did, rejecting Noakes's LCHF suggestion.

Let's summarise: at that point Leenstra had posted a question on a public forum, received different opinions, including from two health professionals – one of them a registered dietitian – and been provided with the contact details of one of those professionals with an invite to get hold of her. Leenstra was free to choose which one to follow up with, and she agreed, publicly, to contact the registered dietitian. Theoretically, things could have stopped there.

However, the day after Ellmer's invite for Leenstra to contact her, Julsing-Strydom entered the discussion and reacted with a tweet directed to Noakes, written thus: 'I AM HORRIFIED!! HOW CAN YOU GIVE ADVICE LIKE THIS??' For those unfamiliar with the idiosyncrasies of social media, the use of uppercase letters is normally reserved to express a strong feeling of annoyance, displeasure or hostility. On its own, Julsing-Strydom's use of uppercase in a tweet is perfectly acceptable; it shows how she must have felt reading Noakes's tweet, and there are possible reasons for that. Firstly, she had a four-month-old daughter she was breastfeeding, so she had a personal as well as a professional interest in the topic under discussion. Secondly, as she would later testify, she had had a strongly worded engagement the previous month with Noakes over what she saw as his dispensing nutritional advice to breastfeeding mothers during a talk. It's easy to imagine that for Julsing-Strydom the tweet was the last straw, and so she submitted her complaint, including screenshots of Noakes's tweet, to Legal Med. The accompanying email read:

'To whom it may concern. I would like to file a report against Prof Tim Noakes. He is giving incorrect medical [nutrition therapy] on Twitter that is not evidence based. I have attached the Tweet where Prof Noakes advises a breastfeeding mother to wean her baby on to a low carbohydrate, high fat diet. I urge the HPCSA to please take urgent action against this type of misconduct as Prof Noakes is a celebrity in South Africa and the public does not have the knowledge to understand that the information he is advocating is not evidence based. It is specifically dangerous to give this advice for infants and can potentially be life-threatening. I await your response. Claire Julsing-Strydom.'

The wording is a little breathless, and the reason for that would emerge in the hearing.

The complaint contains many factors that Legal Med would have considered, but five pertain to focus points covered so far in this book: the limits to the public's understanding of science, in this case that of human nutrition; the complexity and unreliability of academic research behind that science; the media profile of Tim Noakes, and the idea that he is a 'celebrity'; that the complaint related to something said within a disrupted media environment; and the suggestion that nutritional advice is a clear-cut case of right or wrong.

What the legal department would have known when they received the complaint was that the complainant was another health professional; this wasn't just someone with a beef about their proctologist having cold hands. This meant that the complainant would have understood the potential outcomes of submitting her complaint, especially one claiming that an act by a fellow health professional was 'life-threatening'. The fact of the matter is that Legal Med saw sufficient seriousness in the complaint to investigate.

However, inconsistencies in Julsing-Strydom's complaint soon came to light. She supposedly submitted it on behalf of ADSA, and yet didn't make that clear in the complaint. When questioned in the HPCSA hearing that her complaint triggered, she replied that it was the first time she had registered a complaint, saying, 'I was not aware that this email would actually be, you know, used at this level.'

Now, after 30 years of interviewing people for the media, if there's something I've learnt it's that the most honest comments are usually unconsidered – made as an aside, when thoughts are wandering, or if a little flustered. Perhaps, I thought, Julsing-Strydom hadn't really thought through what was going to happen once she submitted the complaint.

Furthermore, a forensic analysis of Twitter timelines and the submission date and time of the complaint shows that Julsing-Strydom publicly expressed her horror on Twitter on 6 February 2014 at 07:48, and sent her email to Legal Med less than an hour later, at 08:47. It's fair to say that Julsing-Strydom was upset when she wrote that email.

Based on the findings of a preliminary committee of inquiry, the legal department of the HPCSA sent a letter to Noakes on 28 January 2015, saying that he was to be summoned before the Professional Conduct Committee of the Medical and Dental Professions Board. The charge against him was attached to the letter, and it makes for puzzling reading: 'That you are guilty of unprofessional conduct, or conduct which, when regard is had to your profession is unprofessional, in that during February 2014,

145

you acted in a manner that is not in accordance with the norms and standards of your profession in that you provided unconventional advice on breastfeeding babies on social networks (tweet).'

It is so badly written that it would send any sub-editor reaching for a stiff shot of whisky, so it was invariably presented in the media thus: 'charged with providing unconventional advice on social media to breastfeeding mothers'.

When I first read the charge, that part about 'social networks' intrigued me the most. Providing advice on a public social media platform is an ethical catch-22 for any clinician: if they provide generalised information, they can be accused of not taking into consideration the specifics of the patient; yet if they ask for specifics, they risk encouraging the sharing of confidential information on a public platform. There's also the ethical conundrum that if they open a consultative dialogue with someone other than a patient, they can be charged with supersession, essentially 'stealing' a patient; and for the HPCSA, that is grounds for discipline. How is that for irony?

I sensed confusion in the poorly worded charge. On a hunch, I contacted the HPCSA and asked for a copy of their guidelines for how registered health practitioners *should* engage with the public on social media – if the HPCSA were charging Noakes because of his use of social media, they'd obviously have the necessary guidelines in place. I received the following reply: 'Kindly note that the HPCSA doesn't have guidelines around how registered health practitioners should engage with the public on social media.' The HPCSA was clearly in unfamiliar territory. I thought it didn't bode well for a speedy, clear-cut course for the hearing; and I was right.

What started on 4 June 2015, and was supposed to be wrapped up in little over a week, would drag on for almost two years, and if its aim was to deliver a swift, unsparing and public reprimand of a dissident scientist, it failed. Instead, it was to be seized by a veteran of media influence. He knew it had all the elements of a good story: a high-profile dissident scientist facing recrimination; the frothy ire of those rallying to support him; the possible overturning of everything we hold true about what we eat; and in the middle of it all, an innocent baby whose life was apparently threatened. Throw in an injured puppy or two, and the media would lap it up. But Noakes had bigger plans: he was going to use the hearing to turn the tables on conventional science, and start what could be a revolution in biomedical research.

Essentially the case against Noakes hinged on two things: whether his advice was 'unconventional', and whether it was backed by any scientific evidence to the point that it could be considered 'evidence-based'. Therefore testimony for the pro-forma complainant (the HPCSA) focused on that which *is* considered conventional – the South African Food Based Dietary Guidelines – as well as supposedly authoritative academic evidence that seemingly debunked the LCHF diet, also known as the Banting diet. The latter was a meta-analysis and systemic review by Stellenbosch University and UCT (and which from now on I will refer to as the Stellenbosch Review, even though it was referred to elsewhere in the media as the Naudé Review, after its lead author, Stellenbosch University academic Dr Celeste Naudé).

The review purported to have examined all relevant research about the claimed benefits of low-carb diets and concluded that these are 'no more effective for producing weight loss than are high-carbohydrate, or so-called isoenergetic, "balanced" diets'. The media release that accompanied the research, released timeously ahead of the hearing, secured strong traction in mainstream and social media; 'debunk Banting' became a well-used trope in headlines covering the research. For a media that considers the only thing better than elevating heroes is bringing them down, this was joyous stuff.

But it was based on misinformation. I read the media release and compared it to the review. There were discrepancies in the supposed outcomes of the review and what the media release claimed. Interpretation by the untrained eye would have focused on the media release, ignoring the fact that it would have been carefully crafted with an agenda in mind. Science journalism 101: All media releases have an agenda.

What I found most interesting was that the authors of the Stellenbosch Review didn't actually refer to Banting or to Noakes. Neither, in fact, did the media release, but it did refer to debunking. The word was carried at the top: 'Findings debunk claims that low-carbohydrate diets result in more weight loss'. Some media reports made their stories more personal towards Noakes, rehashing the trashy epithet 'celebrity professor'. One report claimed that the Stellenbosch Review proved 'Noakes low-carb diet is not healthier'; another went as far as to claim 'New research shows Noakes diet no more than dangerous fad'.

Media interest in the HPCSA hearing was patchy at first, initially focusing on the evidence for the case against Noakes: the dietary guidelines as mainstays of conventional nutrition, and the Stellenbosch Review as the death knell for LCHF. However, coverage kicked up a notch when, on 10 February 2016, Noakes was called to give evidence. He first addressed questions by his defence team about his expertise and skills as a physician and researcher. It was an excellent opportunity to counter the argument that Noakes is not qualified to speak on nutrition, a criticism that has always puzzled me. Noakes has published over 550 papers in total, of which well over a hundred are on nutrition and sports nutrition, and of those papers his h-index – that measurement of academic productivity and impact – is an impressive 45. There are few specialists in nutrition who can boast an h-index that high. That makes him an established authority not only in exercise science, but also on nutrition. His research in this area covers various elements, such as the role of nutrition in ketone body metabolism, coronary risk factors, lipoprotein metabolism, iron deficiency, menstrual dysfunction, increased cholesterol and increased triglycerides in the blood-stream, diabetes and insulin resistance, and low-carbohydrate diets and exercise performance. It's fair to say that after 40 years, Professor Tim Noakes is a specialist in human nutrition, despite what someone with a three-year diploma will tell you.

With the matter of his qualifications out of the way, his counsel turned to the charges against him. They would have briefed him ahead of it, but his testimony – almost two years to the day after the original complaint was made against him – showed that nerves were still raw. He spoke about responding to the HPCSA regarding the complaint and considering the matter sufficiently addressed, and that he thought they'd consider the whole matter 'a storm in a teacup'.

So when he was actually charged, it came as a brutal shock. He said, 'If I had known what the consequences of this hearing were, I would have done anything in my power to stop it happening because of the cost to me personally, to my family, and so on.' At that point he became emotional, referring to the support that he had received from his counsel and his wife, Marilyn, and, before he could go much further, he broke down in tears. It was a crushing moment for Noakes's team, as well as his family, friends and colleagues who had come to support him.

It was also the moment that the media had been waiting for. Within moments, the news was online: 'Tim Noakes in tears', 'Noakes baulks under pressure', 'Tim Noakes breaks down' and 'Humiliated Tim Noakes in tears at banting hearing'. I remember it well.

I felt sympathy for Noakes, frustration with what was happening, and a deep anger towards an increasingly tabloid, judgemental and biased mainstream media with which I was unfortunately associated. My training as a journalist had instilled in me a sensitivity towards the ethical issues of reporting on people under emotional stress; there was little evidence of that in what I read.

However, the real eye-opener was the response to Noakes's breakdown on social media, specifically Twitter: hardly a mention outside of tweets by mainstream media pointing to their online stories. There's a possible reason for that. Social media taps into, and reflects, popular sentiment, often in all its unrefined glory, and if there's one thing that was becoming increasingly clear on Twitter, it was that popular sentiment was behind Noakes. Do an advanced search on Twitter using the hashtags #NoakesHearing or #TimNoakes or #Noakes with other hashtags such #HPCSA or #LCHF to filter out other people called Noakes, and the support for Noakes was clearly overwhelming. It manifested itself in other memes and hashtags, including one in reaction to the charge against Noakes that his evidence for the benefits of an LCHF diet was purely anecdotal and not evidence-based. The hashtag #anecdotalevidence carried pictures submitted by people before and after embarking on an LCHF diet with details of weight loss and reversal of their ill-health conditions. It also steered people towards an LCHF Facebook page where almost 160 000 people were sharing similar experiences. This would shortly balloon to over 370 000.

This rise in popular revolt on social media against the established nutritional guidelines also came with intense criticism of a number of people and organisations, mainly the HPCSA, ADSA, Claire Julsing-Strydom and other dietitians. The criticism of the HPCSA seemed justified. In all my interviews and all my research, I didn't come across a single scientist or journalist –

even those who were critical of Noakes – who had any measure of confidence in, or support for, the HPCSA and the hearing. Criticism of Julsing-Strydom ranged from subtle digs around why she wasn't at the hearing during Noakes's evidence to disparaging personal comments about her.

Shortly after Noakes's breakdown, there was a turning point in the mainstream media coverage: sentiment shifted more in his favour. Possibly because of sentiment on social media, but more probably because, from that point on, Noakes stamped his authority on the hearing. For 40 hours he provided a systematic review of the failures of the current approach to medicine, and the benefits of an LCHF diet for people who were diabetic and pre-diabetic. He drew on more than 4000 pages of notes and nine PowerPoint presentations, with references from top international scientists and institutions. He explained the evolution of the human diet, the diet-heart hypothesis, and the origin of the obesity epidemic, insulin resistance and metabolic syndrome; and he spoke about infant feeding and complementary feeding, and the science of causation. And this was just the beginning of his defence. He had also lined up expert witnesses that would tear into the current nutritional guidelines and the damning Stellenbosch Review.

I caught up with Noakes in May 2016, between sessions of the hearing. Noakes always has a quiet energy about him, fuelled by a self-confidence that respects the boundaries of polite restraint. He neither shouts nor marches into that space in your face where motivational speakers look for a foothold. And he smiles, a lot. But as I sat down to interview him, I sensed an edginess. His finger kept tapping on the table. He was in a fighting mood. 'I'm going to win this case,' he told me. I asked him if his critics in academia were worried about speaking about the hearing for fear of being misquoted or challenged. 'No, I don't think so.' That smile again. 'They're not confident in their opinions, maybe because their opinions have been influenced by outsiders.' He was referring to organisations that fund much of the research *that* he considers protective of the nutritional status quo and harmful to the evolution of science. 'So many doctors have outsourced their brains to the pharmaceutical industry,' he said.

Again, I felt a little uneasy with his provocative tone, but it was in line with a central theme of his argument: that medicine focused on disease *treatment* through pharmacological intervention, instead of disease *prevention* through correct nutrition. If there was a specific intervention in his crosshairs during the hearing, it was insulin: the manufactured version of the hormone normally made by the pancreas to regulate blood glucose levels. 'Let's say I was a diabetologist on the hill [meaning UCT]. I'll only be well known if I've done large clinical trials using insulin in treatment in type 2 diabetics, and we know *that* insulin doesn't work – it makes it worse – but the moment I admit *that*, I will lose my funding.' *Jason Fung had a similar feeling.*

He spoke in bursts, soundbites almost; the result was a slightly disconnected stream of thoughts, strung together on a thread of zeal. 'So many doctors have bought into the pharmacological model, from the professors down, and that's the basis for the attacks on me.'

I asked if these doctors were in a state of denial. 'Absolute denial. It's cognitive dissonance. Obesity and diabetes rates have gone through the roof. Diabetes affects so many different people in medicine. Surely they'd think, there's more diabetes today than what there was 10 years ago; what's going on? What's happened?'

He went on to say how the standard hypotheses behind the dramatic increases in rates of obesity and diabetes suggested urbanisation, overcrowding or a lack of exercise. 'But what about diet?' he asked. 'If you have a look at the biology, it's absolutely

clear; but they can't go that route, because they'd lose everything.'

I was reminded again of previous times when I had seen Noakes
speak, such as that occasion at the Sci-Bono Discovery Centre,
and the passion with which he communicated his ideas. It can
be unnerving for other scientists, but that is exactly what makes
the media reach out to him. There is a downside, of course, and
it's something that I've known for many years as a broadcaster: never
open your mouth when you're emotional – you may say something that you'll regret. I imagined the media crouched in the wings,
waiting for Noakes to drop his guard, say something controversial and spark heated debate in their online discussion forums.
Should he not temper the passion in his tone? 'I see the other
side,' he told me. 'I cannot walk outside this building without
someone saying to me, "You saved my life."'

That didn't help. I had seen so many radio presenters and
celebrities crash and burn because they surrounded themselves
with sycophants. I challenged him on the dangers of being continually told that he's amazing, the risk of becoming disconnected
from the rigours of the real world, of living in an alternative
reality. He shook his head, leaned forward and smiled again
before telling me of his unease when one woman started telling
him how her health had returned to normal by simply changing
her diet, then laid her head on his shoulder and burst into tears.
'I get embarrassed by it, but that's the level of support that we have
in the community. I think that a significant proportion of the population believe what we're doing. We focus on them.'

I shook my head, puzzled with what I had just heard. He had
used the word 'we'. Not 'I'; 'we'. The critical voice in my head – the
soundtrack all journalists should have playing on a loop – wanted
to strip away the zeal and find what he was hiding. There was part
of me that wanted to believe he was driven by some messianic

conviction, and I looked at him for evidence. He looked at me and smiled. I could hear his finger tapping on the table, the energy in him looking for an outlet. I tried to think of my next question, but my mind was racing to make sense of what I had just heard.

But then I got it. For the first time in all the years I had been researching and writing about Tim Noakes, I finally got it: I had spent all this time seeing Noakes as a *scientist*; I had forgotten he was also a *doctor*. He may have eschewed the traditional route in medicine – claiming he didn't have the emotional strength to deal with the potential death of patients – and followed a wandering quest within academia for over 40 years, but something had forced his return to lead a fight for the lives of people he would otherwise have called patients.

This explained the intensity of his language and his willingness to reach out to social media, the nemesis of traditional science. Sure, he wanted to share his knowledge; but, more importantly, he wanted others to reach out to him and share *their* knowledge about themselves as they changed their diet to address their failing health. Collectively they were the living evidence of the success, or failure, of an experiment in nutrition. Critically, though, for Noakes, these weren't figures on a graph; they were real people.

He alluded to key research of which he'd been a part and that was about to be published, and which would emerge in the next session of the HPCSA hearing. It documented the creation and then replication of a successful lifestyle intervention in rural British Columbia in Canada: 'It's not a traditional hypothesis-driven study; it's a study where the inputs were changed slowly and the outcomes were dramatic.' I pointed out that it wasn't a traditional approach to research and could work against him. 'No, this is the new way of medicine. The outcome was to cure the patients; and we did it.' I said it was an unorthodox approach to medical science, combining research with being a doctor. He seemed to find that appropriate: 'Yeah, absolutely.'

If he seemed confident in winning, it was because he revels in criticism. 'When I get criticised, the first thing I do is assume that I am wrong. That's because I am an academic. I have published over 550 scientific papers and every paper comes back with a critique – you're wrong here, you're wrong there. And sometimes the paper's rejected. Being rejected is part of being a scientist.' The result, he believes, is better research, and, in the case of human nutrition, getting closer to the truth.

It's a truth Noakes believes is inconvenient for many senior health professionals, especially cardiologists, who have lined up to keep him in check. I asked him if it was jealousy; academia is rife with it. 'No, it's pharmaceutical pressure on the medical community.' He traces the pushback to his book *Challenging Beliefs*, and the first time he really started speaking about diet. 'I talked about statins, and I think that is what the cardiologists responded to.'

Statins are a class of medicines frequently prescribed to lower blood cholesterol levels; in fact, they are among the most widely prescribed drugs in the world. In the US alone, the statin drug industry is estimated to be worth about $100 billion a year, and, according to Drugwatch, one statin brand – Lipitor, made by Pfizer, and now out of patent – holds the status as the world's top-selling prescription drug of all time. Two things are evident from this fact: firstly, that's a lot of money to be lost if statins were made unnecessary; and, secondly, there's clearly something wrong with the nutritional lifestyle of the average American if it requires such large-scale medical correction.

Noakes isn't alone in taking on statins. In 2011, the US Food and Drug Administration (FDA) published the first of its warnings against statins, linking them to liver injury, memory loss, type 2 diabetes and cardiomyopathy (disease of the heart muscle).

Since then there has been a raft of lawsuits against the manufacturers of statins.

Noakes quickly moved on to how the Stellenbosch Review had originally been covered in the media: 'The paper was released and claimed the LCHF diet was dangerous. It never showed that. It showed the diets were identical, and we know why.' He smiled and teased to what he had uncovered in the methodology, saying everything would come out at the next session of the hearing. And then his demeanour changed. He shook his head, as if playing a picture over in his mind: 'And these are scientists; how can they spin it like that?' Then, like a fighter returning to his feet, he bounced back: 'It's manipulated science. No, it's not science; it's commercially driven bullshit.' It's rare for Noakes to swear; he was clearly hurt. I closed my notebook and we shook hands. As he accompanied me to the door, he smiled and promised me that the next HPCSA hearing session was going to be a cracker.

On Monday 17 October 2016, the hearing against Tim Noakes continued, with him providing evidence from the Canadian study he had spoken about, and which had been published in the *South African Medical Journal* two months before. He explained how, in 2010, a single lifestyle intervention study, led by former South African physician Dr Stefan du Toit and Canadian epidemiologist Dr Sean Mark, of obese people with diabetes in a rural primary-care practice had grown, despite limited resources, to four other rural practices. In the end, a total of 372 participants, mainly women with an average age of 52 years, were tracked and evaluated in terms of changes in certain health indicators while following a strict LCHF diet. The participants lost an average of 12 per cent of their initial body weight as a result of the intervention, but, more importantly for Noakes, the prevalence of metabolic syndrome dropped from 58 per cent at baseline to 19 per cent at follow-up. In fact, all participants showed signifi-

Again, possibly cholesterol levels do not matter, unless they are "really low" or "really high".

2019-04-10

cant improvements in their cardiometabolic profiles – their risk of diabetes, heart disease or stroke – to the point that they were able to significantly reduce their use of hypoglycaemic, antihypertensive and cholesterol-lowering medication. Noakes summarised this research with his characteristic flair for the dramatic: 'This is an irreversible condition, and we reversed it by putting these people on the diet that we are told is harmful.' And if that wasn't clear enough: 'The high-carbohydrate diet that these people were originally eating was the cause of their metabolic syndrome; that is what this data proves.' He wasn't finished: 'And all the people who have complained about me over the last five years, not one of them has evidence that their diet is healthy. Not one has done an intervention trial; but we have, and it works.'

2019-04-10

The science establishment may have rebuffed the data, but the story of a small team of physicians and scientists doing research on a shoestring budget in the wastelands of Canada and dramatically reversing chronic health conditions found traction in the media. One of those to pick up on the story was Jerome Burne, an award-winning veteran of British health and medicine journalism. In an article published on 22 August 2016, titled 'Radical doctors throw away rule book to beat diabetes and obesity', he wrote: 'This initiative comes from a self-styled "rag-tag" band of clinicians and data geeks in Northern Canada who have thrown away the rule book and started from scratch. Questioning the official guidelines, they have begun gathering evidence on what does work in the real world.'

'Real world'? I liked that.

When it came to cross-examination, the media in the room again bristled with excitement. There was the expectation of another Noakes in tears; but they were to be disappointed. The Noakes who now faced a barrage of questions showed little evidence of crumbling; in fact, he seemed to grow stronger in his resolve and, like a seasoned Test batsman, relished the opportunity to parry any charge. He often used questions by the HPCSA's advocate, Ajay Bhoopchand, to provide further evidence supporting his own case. For example, when Bhoopchand focused his cross-examination on Twitter, insisting it was an 'inappropriate forum' for doctors to give out any medical or nutrition-related information, Noakes countered with the correct observation that the instant, frank and public corrective-feedback mechanism of Twitter doesn't exist in conventional private consultations between doctors, dietitians and their patients.

If Noakes secured a coup, it was in the specialist witnesses who rallied to his call and bore into the foundations of the case against him: the dietary guidelines and the Stellenbosch Review. Zoë Harcombe was one of those specialists. Harcombe embodies the maxim that dynamite comes in small packages. Slight of build, demure and softly spoken, with a characteristic British penchant for measured expression, Harcombe hides a veritable arsenal of insight into not only dietary guidelines, but also the research and methodologies used to shape them. She has a doctorate in public health nutrition, and her area of expertise is the randomised controlled trial and epidemiological evidence for the introduction of US and UK dietary-fat guidelines. She especially enjoys picking apart data in meta-analyses and evaluating them against systematic reviews. Harcombe is a Sherlock Holmes of scientific statistics.

Harcombe started by tackling the methodology of Ancel Keys and his Seven Countries Study, the bedrock of US and other countries' dietary guidelines. Like other data specialists who have since examined the study in detail, Harcombe discovered basic errors that suggest Keys was either sloppy, biased or forgetful. She also presented one of the most damning testimonies against the guidelines: obesity rates in the US and the UK began climbing in

both countries after the guidelines were introduced, in 1977 and 2019-04-10
1983 respectively.

Harcombe then testified that her examination of the Stellenbosch Review uncovered some anomalies, including the use of studies that failed the review's own inclusion criteria, and therefore risked distorting the outcomes; the use of invalid and subjective meta-analysis subgroupings; and the extraction of data that was, in her words, 'repeatedly inaccurate' and 'inexplicable'.

Harcombe also testified that there was nothing really LCHF in a number of the diets that were tested. The average dietary intake for 14 of the studies included in the review was 35 per cent carbohydrate, 35 per cent fat and 30 per cent protein. That's pretty even. A genuine LCHF diet is very different; it's normally between 5 and 10 per cent carbohydrate and 80 to 85 per cent fat; that's very uneven. As Harcombe summarised, they couldn't judge LCHF diets 'because they didn't study them'.

I caught up with Harcombe after her testimony. I was intrigued as to why she was willing to fly all the way from the UK to deliver testimony for someone she didn't know that well 2019-04-10 (it must be noted that Noakes personally covered the costs of 2019-04-10 those who provided testimony on his behalf; no payment was Good to note. made by The Noakes Foundation). Harcombe first heard about 2019-04-10 Noakes from her brother-in-law, an endurance athlete, who had dramatically improved his performance by following Noakes's guidelines around fluid intake and an LCHF diet. 'Then I got the opportunity to present alongside "The Prof" at the February 2015 LCHF conference in Cape Town and realised how brilliant he is.' She said she was astounded at the shocking treatment being 2019-04-10 meted out to Noakes: 'What on earth is South Africa doing putting their most brilliant A1-rated scientist on trial for? They should be putting him in charge of public health!'

She spoke of her love of raw data and distrust of broad policy

statements made by public health bodies that interpret that data.
I offered the 'Sherlock Holmes of scientific statistics' title I had
scribbled in my notebook with a question mark next to it. She
seemed to like it, especially because someone else had used a similar description when reviewing her book *The Obesity Epidemic:
What caused it and how can we stop it?* 'I love numbers,' she
added, deflecting credit with typical British modesty. She was less
courteous towards the Stellenbosch Review. I needed context, so
I asked her whether she had encountered similar anomalies in
other meta-analyses and systematic reviews she had studied. She
was blunt: 'No, I've not seen this number of errors previously.'
She reminded me of how she had described the review in her
testimony: 'personal, unprofessional and flawed'.

That was strong language. I had to find out if it had any merit,
so I contacted Celeste Naudé, the lead author of the Stellenbosch
Review. Naudé is Senior Researcher at the Centre for Evidence-
based Health Care (CEBHC), a coordinating and directive institution for research and training in the field of evidence-based
health care, at the Stellenbosch University Faculty of Medicine
and Health Sciences. She said that there was nothing personal in it:
'This review was no different to any of the other independent
systematic reviews and evidence appraisals that we do at the
CEBHC if approached by knowledge-users who need to better
understand the body of evidence around a particular question
or questions.' It was the 'knowledge-users' that interested me.
I asked her who funded the review. She told me the South African
Medical Research Council and the Effective Health Care Research
Consortium, which is funded by the UK government's Depart-
ment for International Development.

Funding for research, as we know, is important, but it does
raise ethical issues around potential influence and conflicts of
interest. Naudé denied that this was the case with the Stellenbosch

Review. 'The funders had no role in either study design, data collection and analysis, decision to publish, or preparation of the manuscript; and the authors weren't financially conflicted; and the findings of the review in no way directly influenced their funding or salaries.' She clarified that they did not receive funds from any commercial organisations that could directly or indirectly benefit from the question addressed by the review or its findings.

Naudé then suggested something that I thought odd. She said she was surprised that the review was used in the case against Noakes: 'Yes, it was a key piece of evidence; however, this was unexpected, as the review has little, if any, relevance to infant nutrition, which was the topic of the complaint and subsequent HPCSA hearing. In contrast, the review is relevant to overweight and obese adults.'

If Zoë Harcombe had scared the HPCSA, a nightmare was waiting in the next witness: science investigative journalist Nina Teicholz, who backed up exactly what Harcombe had said about the nutritional guidelines, but went even further. Drawing on her decade-long research behind her book *The Big Fat Surprise*, she showed how the machinations of a cabal of scientists with political influence and a penchant for research that only supported their hypotheses gave birth to the US Dietary Guidelines, which have since become entrenched around the world. She echoed much of the testimony already presented, which showed that the science behind Ancel Keys's diet-heart hypothesis was deeply flawed. As Teicholz put it, 'If you read 10 000 nutrition papers, as I've done, they all telescope back to Keys's Seven Countries Study.' It's ground zero.

Step by step Teicholz provided evidence showing that what we now consider 'conventional advice' on nutrition is based on faulty science; as a result, it is detrimental to most, and dangerous to many. The implication was that the opinion _that_ Noakes had presented to Pippa Leenstra on Twitter was technically, academically and medically in line with the growing scientific evidence that showed the benefits of an LCHF diet, especially in the treatment of obesity and diabetes.

Importantly, with respect to a key component of the charge against Noakes, Teicholz explained how successive studies – including those in Africa – have shown that feeding young children food high in fats helps convey important fat-soluble vitamins, such as vitamins D, E and K, which in turn contribute to healthy growth. This meant that current official dietary advice, which encourages low fat, could deprive weaning infants of the mechanism needed to absorb vitamins and other nutrients during their most formative years. Cross-examination of Teicholz by Advocate Bhoopchand withered to a few questions. Teicholz later told me that Bhoopchand even called her over to his table afterwards and asked her to autograph his copy of _The Big Fat Surprise._

Watching Teicholz during testimony, I sensed that she wasn't there to support Noakes personally – they didn't seem to be friends. So I asked her why, like Harcombe, she had been willing to fly thousands of kilometres, without any payment, to give evidence at a hearing – not the most pleasant of experiences – for someone she hardly knew. 'I came to stand up for the science,' she replied. 'I believe that the science on low-carbohydrate nutrition has been suppressed and attacked and ignored, and that the dietary guidelines used to defend the persecution of Tim Noakes and others is not based on sound science.' She went on to explain how, like Noakes, she had been persecuted for standing up for science, 'so I feel that those of us who are sticking our necks out for science need to support each other'.

I confirmed that this was the first time _that_ she had actually met Noakes, and that, like Harcombe, most of what she knew about him was what she had read. 'I didn't really know about his work in sports science and sports nutrition. I just knew that he was highly regarded in his field, an A1-rated scientist.' I asked her for her impressions now that she had met him. She smiled, seemingly a little surprised by what she had discovered: 'He's a lovely, gentle man. He seems to be a very kind and modest human being.' Perhaps she had expected someone more terrier-like?

'I had expected him to be more of a crusader, a self-promoter, because that's the way he's been portrayed. But I didn't find that at all. He was so modest, almost embarrassed about his fame. When you walk down the street, you can't go 10 feet without someone shouting out, "40 kilos, professor!" "15 kilos, professor!" – referring to how much weight they've lost while Banting. In every hotel and restaurant we went to, people knew him. In South Africa, he's a complete rock star, beloved. But he doesn't bask in it or appear to seek it. He was really far more of a modest academic type than I'd expected.'

I took this opportunity to explore further Teicholz's research into the pushback against health professionals like Noakes; I asked her whether she thought the hearing was evidence of that. It was an unfair question, but I felt it needed to be asked. She was circumspect. 'You can only speculate what the motivations are, but what you see happening in South Africa and elsewhere around the world is attacks on people who have spoken out on the science of carbohydrate restrictions. Authorities have threatened to take licences away from dietitians, doctors and other health-care professionals who are counselling carbohydrate restriction in places like Australia and New Zealand.' Here she was referring to the likes of Gary Fettke and Jennifer Elliott. 'Tim Noakes is part of the same effort. There seems to be an effort to suppress the scientific literature on low-carbohydrate diets, as well as those who are promoting them.' She paused as if to reflect. 'So, yes, I see this as an effort to suppress Tim Noakes and the science that he is trying to speak out about.'

Teicholz's current research is showing evidence that the US Dietary Guidelines Advisory Committee buried a sizeable body of scientific literature on the safety and efficacy of LCHF in their most recent report. 'There are more than 74 RCTs [randomised controlled trials] on thousands of people showing that the low-carb diet is safe and effective, yet this evidence was actively ignored by the expert committee.' According to Teicholz, as this information comes to light, there's likely to be a gradual swing in favour of those who, like Noakes, are encouraging a re-examination of what is considered conventional wisdom around nutrition. In the UK, for example, there's a very strong movement for LCHF, but there's also vigorous pushback. For Teicholz, things are getting quite heated. 'There are basically diet wars breaking out all around the globe.'

If this were the case, Marika Sboros would be at the front line. Sboros is a veteran health journalist and the editor of Foodmed.net, the only media outlet that covered every day of the hearing against Noakes. After a 40-year career in newspaper journalism, 30 of those years spent writing on health and lifestyle, Sboros decided to focus on a media format that allowed her to present research on health and nutrition science, in her words, 'independently of any vested interests, advertisers and lurking editors'. The main aim of Foodmed.net, she told me, is to 'balance the insidious influence of food and drug industries worldwide on health and nutrition advice and to focus on evidence-based health approaches that truly aim to "first do no harm"'.

Perhaps this was the reason that Sboros dedicated an entire section to a day-by-day breakdown of events at the hearing. It must have been a labour of love; she has certainly received no payment for it. I asked her how she would have pitched the hearing to an editor.

The journalist in her kicked in: 'I don't think that it's hyperbole to describe it as the Nutrition Trial of the 21st Century.' How would she support that claim? She didn't blink: 'This hearing has global implications for the science of nutrition, and the science – or more likely lack thereof – on which our official dietary guide-lines are based. It also goes to the heart of freedom of expression, especially for scientists – something that our constitution guarantees.' There was more: 'It's also an attempt by powerful vested interests to stifle scientific debate, and discredit a famous scientist because of the threat that he represents to them.'

I challenged her on the tone of her coverage. It seemed decid-edly pro-Noakes; she certainly had little of worth to say about the HPCSA. 'I think that the HPCSA is a patsy in this case – I don't think the HPCSA legal staff in this case have any idea of how they are being used and by whom.' She listed those whom she thought were guilty: doctors, especially cardiologists and endocrinologists. And dietitians? I asked. She nodded, then shrugged. 'The dietitians are proxies – witting or unwitting, I'm not sure. What I am sure about is that all these people desperately want to shut Noakes up because he threatens their reputations, livelihoods, funding and income streams from sponsorships. And because in many cases they just don't have the courage to admit "I got it wrong".'

Her research backed up evidence presented by Teicholz: 'Behind them stand the powerful food and drug industries. I don't think that it is coincidence that all the doctors and dietitians involved in this case have links to food and drug industries directly or indirectly.'

She dismissed any suggestion that she was a Noakes cheer-leader. 'When I first attended the hearing, I thought that Noakes was paranoid.' So it wasn't just me, I thought. 'But eventually I came away convinced that he was clearly onto something.' Her journal-ism instinct kicked in and she stayed on and followed the evi-dence: 'The more I dig, the more I am appalled and fascinated in that equal measure at what these top doctors and academics in South Africa have got up to just to muzzle and demonise one man – a brilliant and ethical one at that.' That sounded a bit like cheer-leading; perhaps a bit biased? 'Sure I'm biased,' she replied, 'but in favour of good science. Anyone show me solid science that he's wrong, and I'll happily write about it.'

I was interested how a former newspaper editor judged the coverage of the hearing in the mainstream media. Sboros is slight in build, almost elfin, but bristles with a steely temperament born from years of combat in a competitive newsroom. She lashed out: 'In my honest opinion, mainstream media mostly covered the hearing badly from the start – hardly giving it any coverage, and, when they did, it was amateurish, lacklustre, with little context, often gratuitously nasty.'

She said it was much like coverage of Noakes in the years before the hearing, where reports were inflammatory and defamatory, with little or no research behind them. I was surprised with that, because I had seen little evidence of it when I examined the media archives Noakes had donated to UCT. I made another note to ask him if he had just kept the good stuff. *Good to ask.*

Sboros affirmed what I remembered of the coverage in the lead-up to the hearing. 'One reason I started interviewing Noakes from the outset in early 2014 was articles I read suggesting that he had gone mad, lost the scientific plot, was a danger to the public, and would soon be committing genocide. I read one long magazine article by a young journalist I respected who quoted Noakes throughout directly. It turned out that the journalist hadn't ever spoken to him! When journalists did speak to him, they still misquoted him. That whet my appetite.'

If there was something Sboros did notice, it was the tone in the coverage as the hearing progressed. 'It was more informed and balanced. Interestingly, the positive articles far more outweighed the negative ones. And his critics were silent. That's probably because of the compelling science that emerged.' She also had a reserved praise for the role that social media played in covering the hearing, especially in exposing articles by journalists who were biased and scientists who didn't do proper research. 'To me, the Noakes case is a brilliant example of the wisdom of the crowd successfully challenging the "wisdom" of the Anointed.'

I left Sboros confident that I had tapped into a representative sentiment of those in the media who supported Noakes. Now I needed to cross the floor. Finding people in the media who were critical of Noakes was challenging. Many online articles didn't carry a byline, and those on social media, who made no attempt to hide their vitriol towards him, hid behind noms de plume and avatars. No, I needed someone unafraid to challenge Noakes openly, someone who could be expected to provide a cogent line of reasoning, and without resorting to truncated words and emojis. This meant speaking to someone who incensed Noakes, and who is intimately connected to the very beginning of my investigation.

His name is Jacques Rousseau, and if Noakes and his supporters have a nemesis, it is he. A lecturer in logic at the Faculty of Commerce at UCT, he is also the son of Jacques Rossouw – Noakes's opponent at the Great Centenary Debate – even though the spelling of their surnames is different. I considered that a private matter. Rousseau had been writing about Noakes long before the hearing, and his blog, Synapses, had already developed a reputation for its highly critical analysis of Noakes whenever he was finding traction in the media.

I spent some time reading what Rousseau had written about Noakes and picked up a thread of an argument. But there was something else that I hadn't expected. Intrigued, I arranged to meet Rousseau, who seemed completely comfortable with the idea of chatting with me. We met at a sunny outside café overlooking

Mouille Point in Cape Town, one of the few places in the city that would allow him to smoke and drink coffee. Given Rousseau's background in philosophy, it seemed a suitably contemplative setting.

I got straight to the point. 'What is it about Tim Noakes that you have an issue with?' He thought for a second and said, 'He talks about how we ignore the evidence, but then does the same; and if you point these things out to him, he simply blocks you on Twitter and calls you a troll.' He dismissed Noakes's claim that he was his father's proxy: 'I have never expressed a view on the LCHF diet, or the science of the diet. That's why the thing about my father is a red herring. My father is a scientist; I'm a logician. I write about the arguments and the logic and the hyperbole of Tim's expressions; I don't write about the science of the studies – I don't know enough to write about the science or the studies.'

That, for me, was an important point. Generally, most of the argument against Noakes – at least that which was coherent – centred on the science of the debate, something that was unlikely to be settled any time soon. This was different; it was more about the messaging. But first there was an issue I needed to get out in the open: that element of Rousseau's writing that I hadn't expected, where he seems to support Noakes. Rousseau nodded. 'I've made the point that he may well be right, and that I hope he's right, because it's a nice, elegant solution to all sorts of disease and public health burden expenses and so forth.' He seemed bemused by my surprise. 'Here I think is where people who are more vociferous critics of Tim than I am get things wrong, because they say he is a narcissist or chasing glory or chasing the money or a Nobel Prize, whatever it might be. I think he's trying to help people, to eliminate a public health crisis, or at least mitigate against a public health crisis, and that his motivations as a physician are intact. He wants to heal people in a sense.' Okay, now I was confused. 'He's certainly a slick operator in terms of public relations and so forth,' Rousseau continued, 'but I don't think that it's ego that fundamentally drives it.'

Back to the messaging; I believed that this was a key component of Rousseau's objection to Noakes. I was right, and it seemed to be tied to Noakes's belief that sometimes conventional wisdom needs to be completely overturned. 'There's a greater value in my mind to defending the scientific method,' said Rousseau. 'While what Noakes is saying may end up revealing something fundamental that'll transform the way we eat and the way we live, treating this in a way that respects the basic tenets of how science is the slow incremental process of building up or rejecting all hypotheses, of building new ones, etcetera, is worth preserving. If you are an A-rated scientist as in his case, you should have a motivation to defend that scientific method as well, and defend sober scientific reasoning; so it doesn't suit that virtue or goal to be telling people in absolute terms that you will not get diabetes or cancer if you follow the LCHF diet. That's an example of a hyperbolic, evangelical statement, not of a scientifically responsible or sober statement.' I sensed in Rousseau an element of disappointment in Noakes, rather than remonstration; but I could've been wrong.

If I had found a nerve, it only seemed right to tweak it. Was it perhaps not so much about Noakes's challenging of convention than the way he was doing it in the public space? 'That is a major issue. There are two aspects. Firstly, the standards of scientific reasoning that he supports; and that would be true whether it were in the public domain or not. If it were in the academic arena, then I think peer review might take care of a lot of it; people would say that's not good evidence and he wouldn't get a lot of this stuff published if it were in academic literature. So one could say that this is one way of avoiding the scrutiny of one's peers. He is publishing some stuff, but it's not as if he is doing most of this work in academia – he's doing it in the public domain. So he's avoiding the ordinary scrutiny of academia. The second issue is that he's teaching people a profoundly dangerous idea that truth is resolved through democratic processes. This whole "wisdom of the crowd" thing.' Rousseau then referred to 'the professoriate of the Twitterati', a term he had used in a column in which he challenged the idea of combing Twitter users for data that could be used in some form of meta-analysis. 'Noakes's idea is that thousands of anecdotes add up to facts. That avoids the scrutiny of your academic peers. He's teaching people bad epistemology – that truth is resolved through consensus.'

Rousseau had hit upon a point that will spur fierce debate within academia in the future: whether scientists should use new technologies within social media to gather information that could be used as research data, essentially disrupting the entire scientific method. Think the randomised-controlled-trial equivalent of Uber.

Seeing as the issue of Noakes's use of Twitter had been a key component in the HPCSA's charge against him, I had to ask Rousseau if he thought that Noakes was influenced by the comments from his thousands of followers. 'I don't think so; [although] he gets constant validation and that can contribute to the filter bubble and a constant absence of criticism of his point of view.' He added that the ball was in Noakes's court as to where he saw the greater value as a scientist. 'If you assume that he is still that intelligent, scientifically minded man, then one would imagine that the greater influence would be from the literature rather than from Twitter; but if he has become the public evangelist more than the spokesperson, then the balance might shift more towards being influenced by Twitter than by the literature. But insulating yourself from opposing points of view makes it easier to never believe you're wrong.'

Rousseau lit another cigarette, took a deep drag, thought for a while and steered the conversation towards the HPCSA hearing against Noakes. He had another curve ball for me: 'I have defended Noakes regarding the hearings. They're stupid and a silly waste of time, and he did nothing wrong as far as I'm concerned.' I thought he would've welcomed Noakes's public comeuppance. Rousseau dismissed the idea that it was ever going to come out of the hearing. 'The HPCSA looked like a bunch of bumbling fools and he was given 10 days or more to do an exhaustive analysis and promotion of his diet. That should never have been part of the hearings. Noakes very carefully leveraged that into a platform to promote his scientific worldview.' I suspected that he also had harsh words for the alleged forces behind the hearing. Again, I was right. 'There seems to be reluctance for many organisations and dietetic bodies to think outside the box,' said Rousseau. 'They feel threatened; they have a livelihood to protect and a cosy little coterie of government support, and so of course those vested interests are going to lash back against it, and that needs to be interrogated, but I don't think the answer to it is to become equally inflexible.'

There was that thread again, that line of reasoning that seemed to loop its way through Rousseau's writing. I started to believe that I had got to the nub of his problem with Noakes, and it was not just because Noakes's language in the media was perhaps sending a wrong message, but specifically because the issue was around something so important: food, our emotional connection with it, and the issues of social identification and self-awareness. Was Noakes capitalising on this to get coverage in the media? Rousseau seemed to like that line of thought. He lit another cigarette and sat back in his chair. 'Yes, but on the basis of good motives, and I don't have a problem with that. I think on his *that,* own logic he must do that, because it's so vitally important. But when humans are emotionally invested, they're not always entirely rational. They're not always entirely rational in any case, but especially when they're emotionally invested. They therefore become more susceptible to specious reasoning or simplistic reasoning. He as a scientist knows this, so the fault is not that he's using the media to push this message; the fault is that he's exploiting our lack of critical judgement when it comes to things *that* we are emotionally invested in. As much as he cares for our health, he should also care about encouraging us to think critically and carefully about scientific matters, about all science.'

On that I agreed with Rousseau, and as much as it applied to Noakes, it applied to all scientists and health-care professionals, especially in an era of social media, where communications are more numerous and competitive, and, in the words of American political scientist Joseph S. Nye, 'a plenitude of information leads to a poverty of attention'.

I thanked Rousseau and switched off my voice recorder, and we chatted amiably about other issues taking root on the UCT campus. We finished our coffees, shook hands and said our goodbyes; and then Rousseau wished me luck with the book. I believed he really meant it.

I grabbed my notebook and tapped it thoughtfully before putting it in my bag. I now had some charges of my own for Professor Tim Noakes.

Chapter 9

Disruption and reflection

As I stepped from my car into the blazing Cape Town summer, a hot, beery breath wafted over me from behind. I was struck by a sudden sense of déjà vu – I had been here before. Of course I *had* been here before – this was the Sports Science Institute of South Africa and I was here to interview Tim Noakes again – but there was something particularly familiar about it all. I looked at the date on my watch – 7 December 2016 – and did the maths; it was almost four years to the day since I'd first interviewed him for what would become this book.

A lot had happened in those four years, and a lot had changed. Principally, Noakes had been accorded the title Emeritus Professor, meaning he was retired but still affiliated to the university. It also meant more free time to do what he wanted. But it had come with some pain. Those four years had seen him targeted on a personal and professional level in attacks by former colleagues and friends. But in the process he had become the standard-bearer for an increasing number of scientists and health-care professionals challenging what they believed was industry-controlled nutritional dogma.

We sat in the conference room at the Research Unit for Exercise Science and Sports Medicine – he no longer had an office – and chatted briefly about the book. He seemed upbeat and anticipative, but my first question caught him off-guard: 'Do you realise that your Great Centenary Debate with Jacques Rossouw was exactly four years ago yesterday?' I watched his expression. He smiled and nodded slowly, slightly surprised. Perhaps it was the context of time passed, but I was shocked with how much he had aged. We had chatted often since then and I had never noticed it. I followed by asking him if he would have done anything differently, knowing now what had happened.

'Probably not, because I think we're coming to a conclusion that will be very positive for the whole low-carb movement, not just in South Africa, but globally,' Noakes replied. 'And one couldn't have been through all this nonsense without getting there – you had to suffer the pain to produce the outcome.' The term 'sanguine' came to mind.

I asked him about the HPCSA hearing. 'I think that it will be a landmark trial globally in advancing the cause of nutrition science and showing that it has been completely misled and controlled by industry to the detriment of human health.'

Noakes used the term 'trial' purposefully to point out the unintended consequence of the hearing for the HPCSA, that the 'conventional' nutritional guidelines had been put on trial. I immediately thought of the famous 1925 Scopes Trial, where a substitute teacher faced a highly publicised trial for teaching evolution at a Dayton, Tennessee, high school. Noakes explained that it was necessary to use the hearing as a trial to provide evidence that industry-influenced dietary guidelines had fundamentally forced people to change what they ate, and in the process steered them onto a course of obesity and associated ill-health, including diabetes. By doing this in the hearing, Noakes took the matter out of the influence of the medical fraternity and into the open. 'That made the difference. So I regret we had to go through it, but I don't regret the outcome. It was tough for myself and my family, and my wife in particular; but we've come through it and now we're beginning to reap the rewards.' I had met his wife, Marilyn, and was struck by her grace and stoicism, and I understood how those who knew them both well attributed much of his motivation to her unyielding support.

Noakes would reaffirm this later in an email to me in which he clarified the factors behind his brief 'breakdown' during the HPCSA hearing, and in which the media seemed to revel. He explained that it had nothing to do with the effects of the trial on him, Marilyn and his family. It was, in fact, purely out of gratitude to them, and especially to his senior defence team – Dr Ravin 'Rocky' Ramdass and Mike van der Nest – who provided their services at no cost. 'Rocky and I now have an amazing relationship – we truly are brothers – and I have so much incredible respect for him and Mike. It was an expression of love, relief and thanks, not of anything else.'

If there was something else that the hearing forced into the open, it was how the medical academic profession was completely out of touch with social media. They did not understand that it was a public forum for discussion with the power of immediate correcting, or that it was a potentially untapped resource for data that could revolutionise scientific research. I pointed out to Noakes the uncomfortable relationship between science and social media, and he laughed. I challenged him: 'You've suggested that science can benefit from the so-called wisdom of crowds – crowd-sourcing anecdotal evidence that can't be tested, that's supposedly unscientific.' He tapped his finger on the table. 'It's a new way of collecting evidence,' he replied, using this as an opportunity to invoke his rallying cry. 'What's happened is that we have the power of the Anointed – professors and senior academics – and they're all driven by industry and controlled by vested interests who have to sell products. They make patients customers rather than curing them.' A great soundbite, I thought. He waited as I scribbled in my notebook, then continued: 'That's the history of medicine since I've graduated. We are doctors looking after customers and not trying to look for cures. But with social media, the cures are out there.'

He was referring to the ability of people to share their health stories with others. There was a catch, and he knew it: 'Of course, they are anecdotes, but when you have tens of thousands of anecdotes, it's no longer purely anecdotal.' He was challenging the old research mantra 'the plural of anecdote isn't data' by high-lighting a new normal: the power of the collective voice rallying around a call. 'Without social media and all the reports of people turning their backs on conventional nutrition, and in the process curing their condition, this wouldn't have happened. And this is what's broken the back of the cover-up. Without social media and all the reports of people being successful, none of this would have happened.'

For Noakes, the popular groundswell of feedback on social media was not so much an anecdotal reservoir as a Black Swan event; it was nutrition science's Arab Spring.

But this wasn't thousands of people simply hitting a 'like' button; it was the measurable testimony of people whose health had improved to the point where they had been able to turn their backs on the chronic medication on which they had been physically and mentally dependent. It was the flipside of going cold turkey: kicking a habit and the side effect was feeling better. So unambiguous seemed the outcome that Noakes had been approached by international philanthropists – independent of food and pharmaceutical companies – interested in funding this unconventional approach to research. Noakes was particularly proud of this. 'These are people who have themselves benefitted from improvements in their health on the LCHF diet, driving it; they want us to examine the anecdotes of people who claim they have reversed their diabetes and study them, and examine the biological change, and we're going to show that it is possible.' He smiled again, but it was a wry smile; the research would probably be based at UCT.

I sensed a brittle point around his alma mater and academic home of 40 years: it was also ground zero for much of the push-back against him. Many of his former colleagues bristled at the very mention of his name and considered his challenging of convention opprobrious. I found the paradox particularly brutal. The very university that had justifiably awarded him the highest academic distinction also harboured those who wanted to see the back of him; he was for all intents and purposes an honorary outcast.

He swept aside any ill feelings, returning instead to what he believed would emerge from this new line of research. 'You know, every day someone phones me and says I've reversed my diabetes or I'm not taking insulin any more. How is that possible if our profession says it's impossible? They say you can't reverse diabetes; the only reason they say that is because industry is telling them they need to keep patients as customers. If patients have cures, they'll stop taking insulin.'

What he was saying still worried me, and I suspected it had something to do with what convention had taught me: people who are diabetic need medication, and it's tied to inconsistencies in their production of insulin to regulate their blood glucose. I had a childhood friend who would regularly interrupt the day's play to inject himself; all I knew was that if he didn't do it, he risked collapsing and becoming seriously ill. I had seen it happen once, and the image still haunts me. I thought of him and asked Noakes if what he was saying could be interpreted as encouraging people to change their eating habits and immediately drop their insulin. He shook his head. 'What we advise is that people eat and then measure their blood glucose values,' he said. 'If the meal is high in fat and low in carbs with some protein, the blood glucose will change very little. Hence there is no need to inject insulin. The key driver of the blood glucose concentration is the amount of carbohydrate delivered to the intestine by eating. If you are not eating carbohydrates, your blood glucose level is stable and so you don't need injectable insulin to bring it down. That is the very simple biological truth that physicians promoting insulin prescription refuse to acknowledge. We find that once they are reducing their insulin, they can often go onto metformin, which acts in a different way to insulin. The key in the management of all types of diabetes is to reduce to an absolute minimum the amount of insulin that is needed.'

And if people managed to regulate their blood glucose levels through diet and continued to take insulin injections? That, Noakes replied, could induce hypoglycaemic attacks: 'They are absolutely dreadful experiences and can have a serious outcome, including irreversible brain damage.'

I asked him what he thought of the action taken against Gary Fettke and Jennifer Elliott, the health professionals in Australia who had been silenced. He became angry. 'It shows the distortion of medicine that if they don't agree with you, they shut you up. And that's not how I came into medicine. If we knew everything, we wouldn't have to have new ideas, but you can't shut up ideas and demonise people.' Fettke was a personal friend of Noakes, and I suspected that he had a more intimate knowledge of how Fettke was dealing with the judgment; he shook his head sadly. 'It's had a huge impact on his life. He's emotionally distraught. He doesn't know where the next challenge is coming from. He doesn't know what to say to patients any more.' He went on to quote Fettke, who said, 'I came into medicine to help patients, and all I've done is what I believe will help my patients, and then I get targeted and demonised and publicly humiliated.' Noakes could have been quoting himself. He nodded. 'This is their standard approach – if they don't like what you're saying, they don't say let's debate it in open court and give you an opportunity to say what you want to say; they just publicly humiliate you.' This was why Noakes's shrewd use of the HPCSA hearing to put conventional dietary guidelines on trial was so important for the LCHF movement worldwide.

If Noakes had managed to seize the opportunity to achieve momentum while Fettke and Elliott had withered against the storm, it must have had something to do with his experience with the media. 'Surely,' I asked him, 'that has made you more immune to the effects of public scrutiny than someone like Gary Fettke?' He paused for a while before answering. 'That's a good question. I think it's also because I've challenged other forms of conventional thinking in the past, subsequently been attacked, and won; so I've got that backing.' I thought back to his research into over-hydration in sport, and his very public support for Jake White and Lewis Gordon Pugh, all of which earned him loud reproach for challenging what was at the time conventional wisdom. 'It's very difficult to explain to someone who's never suffered rebuke in the media what it's like. I know just how brutal it can be; you either need a thick skin or an ability to ride out the swings and roundabouts that come with a high media profile. It can turn in an instant; one minute you're a hero, the next it seems that everyone's lining up to take you down.'

Noakes said something else that reminded me of the previous interview, when I had first noticed the doctor in him. 'I think what was so hard for Gary was [that] he was prepared to operate on these diabetes patients – literally cut their legs off – and he's not even allowed to tell them how to prevent the problem? That must be very frustrating for him.' He paused and shook his head, and for a second I saw his shoulders sag. Again there was that deep upwelling of empathy that separated the doctor from the scientist. It reminded me of the moment at the Great Centenary Debate when my interest in Noakes was first kindled.

The connection between doctor, scientist and the media was something that I wanted to explore further, but Noakes pre-empted me: 'Anyone who sticks their head above the parapet is going to get nailed, especially if they're active on social media.' It was a point that I had picked up: challenging convention was part and parcel of science; it was how science evolved, and whereas doing so publicly, especially through the media, earned the annoyance of traditionalists within academia who thought that such things deserved to be debated 'internally', something else had to be behind the seemingly overkill reaction of public censure. Noakes could see my mind playing detective. 'The point is that we're threatening industry; we're not threatening science, because we have the science behind us,' he said. 'It's not a scientific debate; it defers to *ad hominem* arguments, just as it did for John Yudkin.'

My hypothesis was taking a beating. I had supposed that the pushback was largely because proponents of conventional nutrition believed that consumers lacked sufficient critical thinking to balance conflicting information and make a sober judgement – in this case, around their health. 'No,' said Noakes, 'that could be their argument, but it's false. Industry is driving it. And the moment that you stand up to challenge their future income, that's when you get targeted.'

Teaching people schooled in obedience to be cynical of authority isn't easy. I'd argue that being cynical isn't easy; it can be exhausting, but it's something drummed into every journalist. Noakes had some tips: 'If there's a product or any intervention

180

being marketed as a consequence of the study – ignore the study. *2019-04-10*
If the people funding the study will benefit from the outcome of
the study – such as pharmaceutical drug trials – ignore the study.
They're not going to allow anything to be published that will
hurt their bottom line. Also look for the conflicts of interest.'
The latter have to be listed by all authors of a published paper,
and it's one of the first ports of call for a science journalist. It
does, however, assume full disclosure.

There was one other issue about the media on which I needed
to challenge him: the seeming absence of any negative coverage
in the media archives he donated to UCT's Jagger Library. 'I went
through your media archives, focusing mainly on newspapers
and popular magazines, and almost all the coverage was positive; that's either because media sentiment towards you at the
time was generally positive – which I cannot believe – or you only
kept the positive articles. Did you only keep the positive ones?' *2019-04-10*
He smiled and then nodded. 'Yes, I kept out all the negative artic-   *Good to*
les.' I was a little shocked; somehow I had expected complete   *write about.*
transparency from Noakes. He held up a finger to command a
point. 'There's a reason for that.' I was listening. 'I've kept all the
negative stuff because I am using it for a book I'm writing that
focuses on arguments against me. I rejoice in the negative stuff,
not only because that's how you learn, but because that's how
your opponents expose their hands, so you know how to defend
against it.' I made a mental note not to challenge Noakes to a   *2019-04-10*
game of poker.   *Humor.*

I wasn't going to leave it there. I had another hypothesis: in a
disrupted media environment, where inexperienced journalists
had replaced seasoned science journalists, coverage of Noakes
in mainstream media has been affected. I put this to him; his
reaction was immediate. 'Absolutely. Previously, journalists would   *2019-04-10*
come, ask for my opinion and report my opinion as I said it, then
   had   *2019-04-10*

ask someone else for theirs to get a balanced opinion. Now there's
no such balance; it's all completely biased. From the moment
they start writing, they put in their personal bias. So every article
is biased either one way or the other.' He went on to note how
journalists now reach out to his opponents – usually a handful
of the same – for comment, knowing they'll get something injurious to Noakes, without even contacting him for a response.
He shrugged it off sadly. 'The balance has gone.' I nodded and
explained to him that because mainstream media is in competition with social media for the attention of the media consumer,
there is an economic necessity within mainstream media to
eschew balance for tension. As I lecture scientists who hope
to get their work into the media: 'Tension gets attention.'

If there was any shift in balance, it was in the sentiment
towards Noakes as the HPCSA hearing evolved. The wild anticipation of a bloodletting that had fed the tone at the start of the
hearing and earned it widespread coverage had subsided, and in
its place reporting had become more muted and sporadic. Had
he noticed that? 'Oh definitely; and one thing I absolutely noticed
in the trial was the moment I started giving evidence, people
who said there was no evidence for the benefits of the LCHF diet
suddenly disappeared.'

If there was one term that defined much of the coverage of
Noakes in mainstream media, it was 'celebrity scientist'. I figured
he would brush it aside; he's certainly faced more malicious
language. I was wrong; he became agitated. 'I think it's deroga-
tory, because celebrities are by definition Hollywood actors and
actresses,' he chided. 'Scientists are not celebrities. It irritates me.
I'm not a celebrity scientist. I am an A1-rated scientist who just
happens to have quite a high profile.'

I was a little taken aback. 'Surely you can understand why
people say that?' I asked. 'You're often in the media.' He reacted

by pointing out the subtle, but savage, subtext in the word 'celebrity': ego. '"Celebrity" sends a message, "Don't listen to him, he just wants to draw attention to himself", and that's not me. Celebrities are good at being celebrities; I'm good at being a scientist.' I had to ask: 'So what you're saying is that you're not the Kim Kardashian of science?' He laughed.

His claim to a lack of ego is important to note, and it seemed lost in much of the coverage of Noakes in the media, perhaps because it didn't fit a narrative: Noakes doesn't see his role as a sole crusader, so the story is not about him. He sees himself as part of a concerted effort by a collective of scientists, researchers and health-care professionals around the world pushing against an industry-sponsored force with vested interests in retaining a pharmacological model of medicine. If you're looking for an entertaining analogy, think Galactic Empire, Jedi, and Noakes as Obi-Wan Kenobi.

There is, however, an image in that analogy that accurately frames the story: a rebel alliance being pursued by a larger entity intent on their defeat. It has compelled Noakes to use his media profile and his ability to withstand public criticism as a force field to lead the charge. He admits that he's now an activist, but there's a personal reason for that: 'I made errors for 30 years and gave incorrect advice to patients that actively led to their ill-health. And that's why ...' His voice trailed off as if choked by a sense of guilt. He looked down and slowly shook his head. He had dropped his guard, and I could see he was hurting. For some strange reason, he feels responsible for perpetuating what he sees as a lie. It was one of those moments that I imagined few of his opponents ever witnessed – a vulnerability born of self-reproach.

I changed the subject towards where he had found so much support: social media. The smile returned. 'I think that it's astonishing,' he admitted. 'It has driven the change. It's forced mainstream medicine to take note, and that wouldn't have happened for another 30 years.' Yes, I pointed out, but it comes with its unsparing feedback mechanism. He laughed and referred to the example that he presented in the hearing of when he misquoted Churchill on Twitter and was immediately corrected: 'I realised that I had distorted the quote for my own benefit.' It takes a brave scientist to pluck himself from the cloister of academia and expose himself to the slings and arrows of social media, where antagonists lie in wait behind pseudonyms and avatars. I asked Noakes how scientists could communicate their work with sufficient popular appeal and scientific rigour in a disrupted media environment, where the role of the journalist as gatekeeper has been sidelined. He smiled, somewhat sagaciously: 'You have to be honest about what you do, because if you're not you'll be exposed, and that's the key. That's the only reason that I survive – I tell people what's true.'

So social media is a source for good for science? 'I think that it's critical, because there are so many people looking at it, and if the science is false, it will be exposed.' I wondered if that was the reason why, when I lecture communication to scientists, there's a definite antipathy towards social media.

There's a balance to the criticism waiting on social media: the opportunity to see a support base develop. I reminded Noakes that he had a passionate and very vocal following on social media, mainly Twitter, who rushed to his defence if they felt that his reputation had been harmed in any way; but they could be brutal at times. I wondered what his feeling was towards them.

'I don't like anyone to be brutal to anyone else, but on the other hand I've been exposed to a lot of brutality, so I think that it's an eye for an eye,' he paused, 'which I don't necessarily support. But it's a difficult space, and if you're going to get into that space, you must expect to get a bloody nose every so often. Everything has consequences.' I sensed that he wasn't talking about himself. What

184

did he mean? 'When I think back to the trial, the consequences for some people were huge, because they didn't think it through.'

I was a little thrown by his answer, not because of what he said, but by the tone of his voice – it wasn't combative; more sympathetic. I pushed him for clarity. 'By "some people", you mean …?' He looked at me somewhat puzzled, as if the answer was obvious. 'Like Claire Julsing-Strydom,' he replied. 'Her life has been turned upside down.'

I was a little taken aback. If anyone's life had been turned upside down, it was his, and yet here he was showing compassion for the very person who hit the 'send' button on an email that launched proceedings that could end his career.

'Do you feel sorry for her?' I asked. He nodded. 'Google her name and all you get is her connection to me. So she's linked forever to me. I do feel sorry for her.'

Did he believe she regretted submitting the complaint? He thought about it for a while and nodded again before adding, 'But the preliminary committee of inquiry should have stopped that thing and prevented it from going forward.' If Noakes and Julsing-Strydom had a common enemy, it was harboured within the HPCSA. Noakes summed it up: 'They could have saved her all this trouble, but they had an agenda.'

I had tried to get hold of Julsing-Strydom, eventually succeeding in speaking with the communications team that had sprung up to protect her, and getting them to appreciate my urgency to get her side of the story. I even submitted the questions and offered her the opportunity to review what I wrote for accuracy. After numerous emails and calls she ultimately declined, which was a pity. Noakes wasn't surprised. 'She's gone underground,' he said.

This was a good time to talk about the HPCSA hearing. Noakes smiled again. 'What it's failed to do is find me guilty, because they never made a case against me. They never could, because there was no case; so what we did is change the focus from me towards the current dietary guidelines and put them on trial in a legal sense, and that's what made this trial so important; it was the first time that this had happened.'

He made a point of emphasising the impact of Nina Teicholz's testimony. 'She showed that the current US Dietary Guidelines were wrongly formulated and based on faulty science, and therefore not evidence-based.' The fact that the *BMJ* later stood by its decision to publish her article proved particularly injurious to the case against Noakes: it essentially flipped it on its head.

Noakes explained the irony: 'The whole debate in this trial was what is unconventional advice, and we were told that it's advice that's not based on evidence. We showed that the current dietary guidelines are not based on evidence, and are therefore unconventional. This means that if this emerges from the trial, then if your doctor encourages you to eat a low-fat diet, he's giving unconventional advice and you can report him to the HPCSA.' I raised my eyes, somewhat surprised; he shook his head: 'Look, that's not going to happen.'

At that point in the interview something strange happened: neither of us said anything. It was as if the whole topic of the HPCSA hearing had actually become irrelevant. I had no compulsion to ask him any more questions on the matter. So much had been said in the media, and I think that we both had the sense that a job had been done and that now it was time to move on.

So I moved on. 'I've been talking to your critics.' That famous boyish, goofy Noakes smile again, 'Yes?'

I continued, 'And I had a long chat with Jacques Rousseau.' He shifted in his seat. I pointed out that Rousseau had used the opportunity to say some positive things about him, and read out what he had said: that he believed Noakes was trying to help people, to eliminate a public health crisis, or at least miti-gate against a public health crisis, and that his motivations as a physician were intact. But Noakes honed in on the last part of Rousseau's comment: 'A "slick operator"? Why does he say that? He makes me sound like the Mafia. Everything he writes has these negative adjectives.' He was referring to Rousseau's many blog posts about him. The term seemed to bug him: 'It's a back-handed compliment.'

This was the first time that I had seen Noakes get really angry; he usually shows remarkable composure, even under intense pub-lic pressure. His ire was aimed directly at Rousseau: 'I think that his approach is appalling. He's written 29 blog posts about me but never spoken to me once, and never attended any of my lectures; he doesn't even know what I lecture on. I talk about nutrition science and I talk about the science behind low-carb eating. I never tell people that they must follow the LCHF diet. I say that there is the evidence, and this is why it's clear to me why conventional got it wrong. I'm a slick operator? I just tell people the facts in a way that they like to hear them.'

Noakes's reaction showed sensitivity towards what he con-siders disrespect. In all our discussions, if there's something that was clear, it was his willingness to engage in debate, to evaluate any evidence presented to him and continually re-evaluate his position with respect to that, as long as it was done within the parameters of respectful engagement. That respect should be accorded to his position as a leading scientist and his integrity as a doctor. Indeed, days after our interview, Noakes contacted me, clearly still bothered by Rousseau's comment. 'I am not happy with this "slick" term,' he said. 'I am not slick. I am honest and people respect that honesty, since it is in such short supply these days.'

Back in the interview I honed in on Noakes's reaction to

criticism. 'Rousseau says that you complain about people ignoring evidence but do the same, and when people point that out to you, you block them on Twitter.' He knew *that* Rousseau was referring to himself: 'I blocked him because he was obnoxious. He was not interested in debate, but only in making fatuous comments about me. He was highly disrespectful.' Again, that issue of respect. 'If he was really interested in debating, he would have written respectful comments. His were the opposite. Why would I allow him free access to my followers if his only goal was to humiliate me?' He had a point.

Rousseau had alluded to a criticism of Noakes that others had mentioned to me: that he seems to relish his maverick status and is quite comfortable with the notion that science often needs a serious shake-up. Noakes dismissed this, as well as Rousseau's insistence that the integrity of science is bound up with the slow incremental process of building up or rejecting all hypotheses: 'That's utter nonsense. He needs to read about paradigm shifts – they don't come easily and quietly, because they are so revolutionary. They overthrow the convention, and that is never going to happen by keeping everyone happy.' I thought back to Albert Einstein, Ignaz Semmelweis, Lynn Margulis, Bennet Omalu, Barry J. Marshall and J. Robin Warren. Cases in point, I thought.

While I had allowed myself a moment's pondering, Noakes had continued laying into Rousseau: 'He's really not in a position, either by training or intellect, to really understand what this is all about. Or else he can't extract his own ego from the debate.' His use of the term 'debate' intrigued me. It summoned up threads and images of Noakes's Great Centenary Debate four years earlier, but with Rousseau's father. I put to Noakes that Rousseau had dismissed the idea that he was carrying a torch. 'No, he absolutely is a proxy for his father,' Noakes insisted.

In our interview, Rousseau had used 'filter bubble' to describe

2019-04-10

Two(?) days ago, I deleted someone from my phone contacts, because of his criticism of me. Possibly he was unhappy or liked to criticize people.

2019-04-10

2019-04-10

2019-04-10

188

Noakes's intellectual standpoint. He was essentially saying that Noakes only read what affirmed his beliefs, and listened to what he wanted to listen to; and that the feedback he got from his followers on social media served as an echo chamber. Noakes laughed off the idea: 'That's activist jargon. And that's a key feature of Mr Rousseau' – he emphasised the 'Mr' – 'he sets himself up as the expert in critical thinking, but he has no PhD, he has no scientific publications, he's done no scientific research, he's never put in an application for a grant for money. He targets me because he is part of something directed by his father, himself and the Heart and Stroke Foundation of SA. Don't you worry, I will deal with Mr Rousseau fully in the book.'

He started tapping his finger on the table again; I had a feeling I wouldn't have to wait for the book. I was right. 'What Rousseau's done so successfully is to present himself as a critical thinker, therefore he doesn't need to know anything,' Noakes continued, 'just go through a thinking process, and that I'm not a critical thinker because I do x, y and z. But that's not the point. If you want to be successful in science, you have to see the total picture, and sometimes you have to break the rules because the rules don't work.'

It was at this point that Noakes returned to what he believes will fundamentally change science: the hive of information in swathes of anecdotal evidence available on social media. 'And yet science says, "Oh, anecdotes are not important", he added. I could see his passion rising, he was bristling with energy. He leaned forward, the gentle tapping now a machine-gun-like staccato: 'When you see patients and they speak to you and they tell you what the outcomes are, and you can see them; and then you read the literature and it conflicts the patients' personal experiences, then you have to consider that maybe the literature is wrong; and we know through the work of John Ioannidis that

189

most medical research is wrong.' He paused to compose himself. 'So if you're going to say I'm an echo chamber and only listen to my patients and anecdotes and my own personal experience, well, that's the most valuable information you can get.' He smiled with bemused disbelief. 'But Mr Rousseau ...' he shook his head, '... and he sets himself up as an expert?'

I changed tack back towards criticism levelled against him, not only by Rousseau but also by other scientists who felt uncomfortable with the passionate tone of his language. I suspected this was the outcome of meeting so many people who had seemingly benefitted from shifting to an LCHF diet. 'That could be true. I do say things under pressure; but I get so frustrated. And no scientist is 100 per cent correct.' He baulked, realising he had, in a way, backed himself into a corner. 'You must be allowed to make some errors along the way.' Too late; I had seen a crack in his case.

'So you could be wrong?' I asked. The smile returned, as did his confidence, and he embarked on what could best be described as a soliloquy: 'I read everything on the topic, and that is the way I get to the truth. You can't hide from the truth. If there are findings that disprove my position I would have to include them. Otherwise I will be proven wrong in due course, and I don't want that to happen. By ignoring any single factor that disproves your theory, you are setting yourself up for failure. A really good scientist listens very carefully to their critics, and when those critics are correct, they incorporate that criticism and change the model they are proposing. That, I have done repeatedly; and that is why I am able to successfully challenge so many ideas and ultimately be proven correct. The reason I am successful as a scientist, is because I listen to criticism.'

I mentioned how Rousseau claimed that Noakes was playing to an audience on social media and in the process obviating the rigours of academia. He almost exploded. 'Here's a guy who has never published a single scientific publication telling me about the scientific method? The arrogance is unbelievable!' He pointed to his peer-reviewed papers on LCHF already published. 'So Rousseau's opinions are not factual. They are what he wants them to be. He is too lazy to find out what is the real truth. But the truth would also be very inconvenient for him and for his simplistic worldview. Maybe he should publish a few scientific papers before he makes high and mighty judgements about real scientists with real publications records.'

Things were getting a little heated, so I thought I'd better throttle back a bit. 'Let's talk further about your fans.' I immediately cursed myself for unintentionally using a term loved by Noakes's critics, but it was too late. 'They're not fans,' he reproached, 'they're people whose lives have been changed by following the advice I gave them. They made a decision and found that it works. And that's what people like Rousseau don't understand. They'll dismiss the people who speak up for the diet as a reactionary army that blindly supports me. They don't understand that, within a week or two, people can tell if the diet works for them.' I could see he was associating 'fan' with 'celebrity'. 'This isn't a Hollywood movie; this is life-changing stuff!'

I had chatted with a number of people who had been chronically ill before switching to an LCHF diet; if there's a term they had all used, it was indeed 'life-changing'. The passion and absoluteness with which they spoke of Noakes and the difference the diet had made in their lives may have been scientifically anecdotal, but it was compelling. It was also central to the seemingly unorthodox belief that health, not intervention, should be at the heart of medicine, or as Noakes summed up in a soundbite: 'The function of doctors is to keep their patients out of hospitals, not send them there.'

I looked at my watch, our time was up. As if on cue, Megan Lofthouse, Noakes's ever-protective PA, poked her head around the door. Before I could get up to go, Noakes encouraged me to stay; he had an ace up his sleeve. 'If there's going to be any pressure on doctors to change their approach, it's going to come from the medical insurance companies,' he told me. 'They're the ones footing the bill for people sent to hospital to treat conditions that could be prevented by a simple change in diet. And the disease that is going to break them is diabetes.' He smiled one more time, seemingly enjoying the irony: 'And it's preventable.'

As I walked through the beery summer heat back to my car, the impact of Noakes's final words began to sink in. I had heard people provide anecdotal evidence – or what they considered 'first-person evidence' – of how a switch to an LCHF diet had reversed their diabetes, but I had never really *listened* to them. Perhaps it was the cynicism that came with being a science journalist that immediately cast doubt on any claims – especially those that were extraordinary – unless they could be supported by rigorous research. Perhaps I was viewing it incorrectly. What if each person was viewed through the lens of a regular journalist – as a source? With that in mind, I registered with a Facebook group called 'Banting 7 Day Meal Plans'. It has over 370 000 followers. With the help of the founder, Rita Fernandes Venter, I posted a message requesting testimonials from people who had reversed their diabetes through the LCHF (Banting) diet. I insisted they provide measurables; simply saying, 'I now feel much better' wouldn't cut it.

I sat back and waited. And then they came, one after the other – remarkable stories of people who had been obese, riddled with disease, and who through a simple, but structured, change in their eating had literally changed their life. Typical was the case of a middle-aged woman who, in October 2013, weighed in at 180 kilo-

2019-04-10 Again, cholesterol levels do not matter, unless they are "very high" or "very low"?

2019-04-10 Good to explain.

grams and suffered from type 2 diabetes, with dangerously high blood pressure and high levels of cholesterol. She was on 500 milligrams of metformin (the first-line medication for type 2 diabetes) twice daily, Ridaq for blood pressure, and simvastatin (a lipid-lowering medication) for cholesterol, plus 65 units of insulin at night and 60 units in the morning. Three days after changing to the LCHF lifestyle, she nearly ended up in a coma because her blood glucose had normalised. She immediately stopped all her meds, and for the last three years her regular check-ups have shown that her blood glucose, blood pressure and cholesterol levels are all healthy. 'And best of all,' she said, 'I have lost 60 kilograms. Still a work in progress, but I'm determined to reach my goal.'

2019-04-10

2019-04-10

Another woman diagnosed with type 2 diabetes collapsed and was in a coma for weeks, thereafter in intensive care for months. 'I had to inject myself with insulin six times a day, and was on oral medication for high cholesterol and high blood pressure.' She started the LCHF diet, and within a year had lost 40 kilograms. She no longer requires medication. What stood out for me in her testimony was her claim: 'I took my health into my own hands.'

2019-04-10

One woman wasn't diabetic but insulin resistant. She wrote: 'I was prescribed Glucophage [a trade name for metformin], which I didn't take; also had chronic high blood pressure. Started Banting 19 months ago at 99.9 kilograms; currently maintaining on 68.1 kilograms, so lost 31.8 kilograms. All health markers perfectly normal with last blood tests. My doc approves of me Banting.'

2019-04-10 Good.

2019-04-10

2019-04-10

"sugar-eater"

that

She was reacting to a particular question had included in my request: How their physician reacted to their improvements on diet alone. Most physicians just seemed happy that their patients were getting healthier; if there were any reports of objections, it seemed to be from cardiologists. That wouldn't have surprised Noakes. One testimonial from a middle-aged man that I found

2019-04-10

2019-04-10

enlightening was that whereas his cardiologist celebrated his return to good health, he made it clear he wasn't supposed to recommend an LCHF diet.

I watched the notifications ring up with every refresh with a mixture of fascination and frustration. Fascination for the people who had dramatically reversed their chronic ill-health simply by changing their diet, and frustration that their testimonies remained inadmissible as evidence to the corpus of current scientific research. If every testimony were a case study and the measurables plotted and analysed as data, they would provide a valuable source of information on the efficacy of an LCHF diet in addressing a whole host of non-communicable diseases, one of the most serious being diabetes. The possibilities for the rapid advancement in scientific knowledge were clear. And yet so many scientists seemed largely disinterested in shifting their thinking, either because of arrogance, a reluctance to reach out and connect, or a need to protect their interests.

All this had been made possible because of a disrupted media space, one where the narrative couldn't be controlled, where ordinary people could publish their opinions about science and nutrition and share their stories, and create a community with a voice. Truth be told, the very idea of that voice being wrested from the discipline of journalism, and disseminated and embraced in all its prejudice, inaccuracy and messiness, grated against my every instinct, but I couldn't deny its burgeoning influence.

I realised then that I had, to a degree, arrived at the answer to my quest; when, at the Great Centenary Debate, I had watched Tim Noakes slump in his seat, his body bowed, that seemingly ever-present smile slip from his face, and I had wanted to know why he was doing this, why he was willing to challenge medical convention to the extent that he was alienating former friends and colleagues.

At that point I scribbled the following in my notebook: ~~2019-04-10~~ 'Professor Tim Noakes's characteristic, unrelenting, dissident approach to science had cast a spotlight on the need to re-evaluate everything that we hold dear about human nutrition. But it had come ~~2019-04-10~~ at a tremendous cost – professionally, his career and reputation had been put on the line, and he had suffered very public rebuke. The media had a hand in both. The measured tone of main-stream media had, over 40 years, gradually developed his profile to give him the leverage to challenge convention. Social media had allowed him to connect more directly with media consum-ers; but its disruptive nature had posed a more serious threat to convention, and convention fought back.'

The HPCSA hearing against Noakes was, I suspect, evidence of this. It wasn't about nutrition; it was about vested interests within a flawed science – one that was fracturing, very publicly, within this highly disrupted media space. And that's why the case against Noakes was, in my opinion, doomed to fail from the very begin-ning. The HPCSA has little, if any, understanding of social media, and yet made that a fundamental part of its case against Noakes. The council doesn't seem to realise that a scientist's tweet isn't a personal diagnosis of a patient; it's a comment in a public meet-ing, and one that demands challenge and further discussion. More importantly, it's in a space where media consumers have access to so much information, and where they should be allowed to make their own decisions. That's why Noakes's comments can't be considered harmful, and certainly not 'life-threatening'.

Furthermore, Noakes neither demanded the exchange of personal patient information on social media, nor did he try to ~~2019-04-10~~ use it to coax a patient from another medical practitioner – both deserving of a charge of 'unprofessional' conduct. He played everything by the book; Noakes is a highly skilled tactician in the use of the media.

Much earlier, the book says that Noakes did not give put his email on Twitter, to have the asker contact him.

And that's another reason why the HPCSA was very wrong if it thought it could crush Noakes by putting him on trial. It was taking on a high-profile and very visible scientist with the personality to challenge convention, the professional will to do so, and the power to impact opinion. The very reason he poses a threat to established interests within the nutrition industry also makes him a formidable foe.

I suspect history will show how Noakes turned the tables on the HPCSA, and used the case to change not only our understanding of human nutrition, especially what is considered 'conventional', but also the way science moves forward. It will show that the real hero of the 'trial' was not Noakes, but everyone who had shared their experience of how changing their diet had changed their lives. And something tells me Noakes would have it no other way.

If Noakes has already succeeded in anything, it is in giving extra impetus to those around the world wanting to challenge the stranglehold of the current nutritional guidelines, which seemed to hold so many people in the grip of serious ill-health. So no one would blame him if he were to step back and let others sustain the momentum in order to spend more time with his family, with his feet up or jogging the tree-lined slopes of his beloved Table Mountain. *Really* retire.

But then a notification came through from Marika Sboros confirming that The Noakes Foundation had received a full grant of R5.6 million to research the reversal of diabetes through an LCHF diet alone. It said that Professor Tim Noakes would be directing the research team, which would include doctors, dietitians and scientists at the University of Cape Town's Division of Exercise Science and Sports Medicine, and that the research 'aims straight at the heart of a powerful vested interest: the medical growth industry of diabetes'.

I couldn't help but smile and shake my head. Retire? I think he's just getting started.

Publisher's addendum

On Friday 21 April 2017, as this book was about to go to print, the *[handwritten: 2019-04-10]* independent professional conduct committee passed judgement in the HPCSA case against Tim Noakes. As part of her 60-page judgement, council chairperson Advocate Joan Adams said that the HPCSA – the pro forma complainant – had not proven on a *[handwritten: 2019-04-10]* balance of probabilities that Noakes had been acting in his capacity as a medical practitioner when he sent the tweet, and that he was presumably acting as an author and proponent of the LCHF diet. She pointed out that Noakes was also found not to have contravened any law, regulation or ethical rule, or that the advice given was unconventional or not evidence based. She added, 'On the facts, this committee finds that no actual or potential harm was proven, or that any information provided on Twitter by the respondent, whether unsolicited or not, was dangerous or life-threatening.' She then announced, 'Professor Noakes, on the *[handwritten: I have seen a]* charge of unprofessional conduct, the majority of the committee *[handwritten: video of this]* found you not guilty.' The following was noted by the large media *[handwritten: part.]* contingent present: 'There was thunderous applause and handshakes all-round as Noakes was exonerated.'

In a media statement afterwards, the Association for Dietetics in South Africa – which had lodged the complaint against Noakes

– said: 'We accept the verdict and we are relieved that the hearing has finally been concluded. We welcome the precedent that this case provides on what we considered unconventional advice.'

Bibliography

Adams, Douglas. *The Hitchhiker's Guide to the Galaxy*. London: Pan Books, 1979

Brockman, John (ed.). *This Idea Must Die: Scientific Theories that Are Blocking Progress*. New York: HarperCollins, 2015

Burne, Jerome. 'Radical doctors throw away rule book to beat diabetes and obesity', *HealthInsightUK*, 22 August 2016

Dawkins, Richard. *The God Delusion*. London: Bantam Press, 2006   2019-04-10

Deer, Brian. 'How the vaccine crisis was meant to make money',   2019-04-10
BMJ, 2011; 342: c5258

Eagleman, David. *Incognito: The Secret Lives of the Brain*. Edinburgh: Canongate, 2011

Elliott, Jennifer. *Baby Boomers, Bellies & Blood Sugars: The Key to Successfully Managing Type 2 Diabetes, Pre-diabetes and Metabolic Syndrome*. Bega: Jeburra Press, 2011

———. 'Flaws, fallacies and facts: Reviewing the early history of the lipid and diet/heart hypotheses', *Food and Nutrition Sciences* 5(19), 2014, pp. 1886–1903

Emlen, Douglas J. 'Alternative reproductive tactics and male-dimorphism in the horned beetle *Onthophagus acuminatus* (Coleoptera: Scarabaeidae)', *Behavioral Ecology and Sociobiology* 41(5), 1997, pp. 335–341

Fischer, Jason, and David Whitney. 'Serial dependence in visual perception', *Nature Neuroscience* 17, 2014, pp. 738–743

Goldacre, Ben. *Bad Science.* London: Fourth Estate, 2008

Goodell, Anita Rae Simpson. 'The visible scientists', *The Sciences* 17(1), 1977, pp. 6–9

———. *The Visible Scientists.* Boston: Little, Brown, 1977

Harcombe, Zoë. *The Obesity Epidemic: What Caused It? How Can We Stop It?* Caldicot: Columbus Publishing, 2010

Hitchens, Christopher. *God Is Not Great: How Religion Poisons Everything.* London: Atlantic Books, 2008

Ioannidis, John P.A. 'Why most published research findings are false'. *PLoS Med* 2(8), August 2005

Kahneman, Daniel. *Thinking, Fast and Slow.* London: Penguin Books, 2012

Lepenies, Wolf. *Between Literature and Science: The Rise of Sociology.* Cambridge: Cambridge University Press, 1988

Mark, S., S. du Toit, T.D. Noakes, K. Nordli, D. Coetzee, M. Makin, S. van der Spuy, J. Frey and J. Wortman, 'A successful lifestyle intervention model replicated in diverse clinical settings', *SAMJ* 106(8), 2016

Nelson, Kevin. *The God Impulse: Is Religion Hardwired into the Brain?* London: Simon & Schuster, 2011

Noakes, T.D., N. Goodwin, B.L. Rayner, T. Branken and R.K.N. Taylor, 'Water intoxication: A possible complication during endurance exercise', *Medicine and Science in Sports and Exercise* 17(3), 1983, pp. 370–375

Noakes, Tim, and Michael Vlismas. *Challenging Beliefs: Memoirs of a Career.* Cape Town: Zebra Press, 2012

Nye, Bill. *Undeniable: Evolution and the Science of Creation.* New York: St Martin's Press, 2014

Oreskes, Naomi, and Erik M. Conway. *Merchants of Doubt: How a Handful of Scientists Obscured the Truth on Issues from Tobacco Smoke to Global Warming.* London: Bloomsbury, 2011

Player, Gary, and Michael Vlismas. *Don't Choke: A Champion's Guide to Winning Under Pressure*. Cape Town: Zebra Press, 2010

Resnick, David B. *The Ethics of Science – An Introduction*. London: Routledge, 1998

Sagan, Carl. *Billions and Billions: Thoughts on Life and Death at the Brink of the Millennium*. London: Headline Book Publishing, 1997

———. *The Demon-Haunted World: Science as a Candle in the Dark*. London: Headline Book Publishing, 1996

Smaldino, Paul E., and Richard McElreath. 'The natural selection of bad science', *Royal Society Open Science* 3, September 2016

Snow, C.P. *The Two Cultures*. Cambridge: Cambridge University Press, 1998

Storr, Will. *The Heretics: Adventures with the Enemies of Science*. London: Picador, 2013

Teicholz, Nina. *The Big Fat Surprise: Why Butter, Meat, and Cheese Belong in a Healthy Diet*. London: Scribe Publications, 2015

———. 'The scientific report guiding the US dietary guidelines: is it scientific?' *BMJ* 2015; 351: h4962

Whewell, William. *The Philosophy of the Inductive Sciences*. London: John W. Parker, 1847

Wilson, Edward O. *On Human Nature*. Boston: Harvard University Press, 1978

Zimmer, Carl. 'Mindsuckers: Meet nature's nightmare', *National Geographic*, November 2014

2019-04-10 I have mostly stopped eating cheese. Possibly I will reconsider.